Lecture Notes in Computer Science   7231

Commenced Publication in 1973
Founding and Former Series Editors:
Gerhard Goos, Juris Hartmanis, and Jan van Leeuwen

W0107693

Editorial Board

David Hutchison
 Lancaster University, UK

Takeo Kanade
 Carnegie Mellon University, Pittsburgh, PA, USA

Josef Kittler
 University of Surrey, Guildford, UK

Jon M. Kleinberg
 Cornell University, Ithaca, NY, USA

Alfred Kobsa
 University of California, Irvine, CA, USA

Friedemann Mattern
 ETH Zurich, Switzerland

John C. Mitchell
 Stanford University, CA, USA

Moni Naor
 Weizmann Institute of Science, Rehovot, Israel

Oscar Nierstrasz
 University of Bern, Switzerland

C. Pandu Rangan
 Indian Institute of Technology, Madras, India

Bernhard Steffen
 TU Dortmund University, Germany

Madhu Sudan
 Microsoft Research, Cambridge, MA, USA

Demetri Terzopoulos
 University of California, Los Angeles, CA, USA

Doug Tygar
 University of California, Berkeley, CA, USA

Gerhard Weikum
 Max Planck Institute for Informatics, Saarbruecken, Germany

Jing He   Xiaohui Liu
Elizabeth A. Krupinski   Guandong Xu (Eds.)

Health Information Science

First International Conference, HIS 2012
Beijing, China, April 8-10, 2012
Proceedings

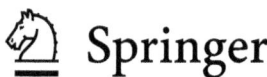 Springer

Volume Editors

Jing He
Victoria University, Faculty of Health, Engineering and Science
School of Engineering and Science, Centre for Applied Informatics
Melbourne City, VIC 8001, Australia
E-mail: jing.he@vu.edu.au

Xiaohui Liu
Brunel University, School of Information Systems
Computing and Mathematics, Centre for Intelligent Data Analysis
London UB8 3PH, UK
E-mail: xiaohui.liu@brunel.ac.uk

Elizabeth A. Krupinski
The University of Arizona, Departments of Radiology and Psychology
Tucson, AZ 85724, USA
E-mail: krupinski@radiology.arizona.edu

Guandong Xu
Victoria University, Faculty of Health, Engineering and Science
School of Engineering and Science, Centre for Applied Informatics
Melbourne City, VIC 8001, Australia
E-mail: guandong.xu@vu.edu.au

ISSN 0302-9743   e-ISSN 1611-3349
ISBN 978-3-642-29360-3   e-ISBN 978-3-642-29361-0
DOI 10.1007/978-3-642-29361-0
Springer Heidelberg Dordrecht London New York

Library of Congress Control Number: 2012934580

CR Subject Classification (1998): H.3, H.4, I.4, H.2.8, I.2, C.2, I.5, K.6.5

LNCS Sublibrary: SL 3 – Information Systems and Application, incl. Internet/Web
and HCI

Typesetting: Camera-ready by author, data conversion by Scientific Publishing Services, Chennai, India

Printed on acid-free paper

Springer is part of Springer Science+Business Media (www.springer.com)

Preface

Welcome to the proceedings of HIS 2012, the First International Conference on Health Information Science, held during April 8–10 in Beijing, China. HIS aims to integrate computer science/information technology with health sciences and services, embracing information science research coupled with topics related to the modelling, design, development, integration, and management of health information systems.

The HIS conference provides a forum for disseminating and exchanging multidisciplinary research results in computer science/information technology and health science and services. It covers all aspects of the health information sciences and the systems that support this health information management and health service delivery. The scope includes (1) medical/health/biomedicine information resources, such as patient medical records, devices and equipment, software and tools to capture, store, retrieve, process, analyze, optimize the use of information in the health domain, (2) data management, data mining, and knowledge discovery (in the health domain), all of which play a key role in decision making, management of public health, examination of standards, privacy and security issues, and (3) development of new architectures and applications for health information systems.

The HIS 2012 program had two eminent keynote speakers, Leonard Goldschmidt from the Department of Veterans Affairs, Palo Alto Health Care System and Stanford University Medical School, USA, and Michael Steyn from Royal Brisbane and Women's Hospital, Australia, one panel discussion on "Medical Devices and Data Processing", and four sections including 15 full papers.

HIS 2012 received 38 submissions from 10 countries and regions. The submissions were carefully reviewed by members of the Program Committee. Based on the reviews, 15 submissions were accepted as full papers. Authors of some selected papers will be invited to submit extended versions to a special issue of the *Health Information Science and System Journal*, published by BioMed Central (Springer). The conference program was of high quality owing to the strong support and commitment of the international Program Committee. We wish to take this opportunity to thank the Program Committee for their dedication and effort in ensuring a high-quality program.

Many colleagues helped toward the success of HIS 2012. They are: Workshop/Panel/Tutor Co-chairs: David Hansen and Guangyan Huang; Local Arrangements Co-chairs: Xiaofeng Meng and Jing Yang; Financial Chair: Jing He; Publication Chair: Guandong Xu; Demo Chair: Chaoyi Pang; Publicity Co-chairs: Haolan Zhang and Huiru Zheng; and Webmasters: Zhi Qiao and Zhangwei Jiang.

We would like to sincerely thank our financial supporters and sponsors. The following organizations generously supported and sponsored HIS 2012: Hebei University of Engineering, Nanjing University of Finance and Economics, National Science Foundation of China, Graduate University of Chinese Academy of Science, and Victoria University, National Natural Science Foundation of China.

Finally, we wish to thank the host organizations, Victoria University and GUCAS-VU Joint Lab for Social Computing and E-Health Research, Graduate University of Chinese Academy of Science, and the local Arrangements Committee and volunteers for the assistance in organizing this conference. The following members helped with the registration, accommodation, and various logistics: Jing Yang, Xun Zhou, Fenhua Li, and Shang Hu.

April 2012   Yanchun Zhang
                                                                 Gultekin Ozsoyoglu
                                                                          Jing He
                                                                       Xiaohui Liu
                                                                 Elizabeth Krupinski

Organization

Executive Committee

General Co-chairs

Yanchun Zhang   Victoria University, Australia
Gultekin Ozsoyoglu   Case Western Reserve University, USA

Program Co-chairs

Jing He   Victoria University, Australia
Xiaohui Liu   Brunel University, UK
Elizabeth Krupinski   University of Arizona, USA

Local Arrangements Co-chairs

Xiaofeng Meng   Renmin University of China, China
Jing Yang   Graduate University, Chinese Academy of Science,
                       China

Financial Chair

Jing He   Victoria University, Australia

Publication Chair

Guandong Xu   Victoria University, Australia

Demo Chair

Chaoyi Pang   Australia ehealth Research Centre

Publicity Co-chairs

Hao Lan Zhang   NIT, Zhejiang University, China
Huiru Zheng   University of Ulster, UK

Program Committee

Guntis Barzdins   University of Latvia, Latvia
Junjia Bu   Zhejiang University, China
Klemens Boehm   Karlsruhe Institute of Technology, Germany
Mihaela Brut   Research Institute in Computer Science of Toulouse,
                       France
Carlo Combi   Università degli Studi di Verona, Italy
Mehmet Dalkilic   Indiana University, USA

Stefan J. Darmoni	Rouen University, France
Fazel Famili	CNRC, Canada
Ling Feng	Tsinghua University, China
Alex Gammerman	Royal Holloway, University of London, UK
Matjaz Gams	Jozef Stefan Institute, Slovenia
Jing Gao	University of Illinois at Urbana-Champaign, USA
Yike Guo	Imperial College London, UK
Bin Hu	Lanzhou University, China
Patrick Hung	University of Ontario Institute of Technology, Canada
Ruoming Jin	Kent State University, USA
Dionisis Kehagias	Informatics and Telematics Institute, Greece
Frank Klawonn	Helmholtz Centre for Infection Research, Germany
Joost N. Kok	Leiden University, The Netherlands
Mehmed Kantardzic	University of Louisville, USA
Ron Kikinis	Brigham and Women's Hospital and Harvard Medical School, USA
Sun Kim	Seoul National University South Korea, Korea
Jie Liu	Beijing JiaoTong University, China
Yongmin Li	Brunel University, UK
Zhiyuan Luo	University of London, UK
Anthony Maeder	University of Western Sydney, Australia
Nigel Martin	University of London, UK
Yuan Miao	Victoria University, Australia
Ruola Ning	Koning Corporation, Lennox Tech Enterprise Center, USA
Yi Pan	Georgia State University, USA
Laura M. Roa	University of Seville, Spain
Hao Shi	Victoria University, Australia
Neil R. Smalheiser	University of Illinois at Chicago, USA
Piotr Szczepaniak	Technical University of Lodz, Poland
Vaclav Snasel	VSB-Technical University of Ostrava, Czech Republic
Jue Wang	Xian Jiaotong University, China
Shuxin Wang	Tianjin University, China
Wang Wenjia	University of East Anglia, UK
Yong Wang	Chinese Academy of Science, China
Zidong Wang	University of Uxbridge, UK
Chen Xin	Nanyang Technological University
Jeffrey Xu Yu	Chinese University of Hong Kong, China
Terry Young	Brunel University, UK
Xun Yi	Victoria University, Australia

Aidong Zhang	State University of New York at Buffalo, USA
Hairong Zheng	Shenzhen Institutes of Advanced Technology (SIAT-IBHE), Chinese Academy of Sciences, China
Min-Ling Zhang	Southeast University, China
Ning Zhong	Maebashi Institute of Technology, Japan
Wenhua Zeng	Xiamen University, China
Xiuzhen Zhang	RMIT University, Australia
Zili Zhang	Deakin University, Australia

Sponsoring Institutions

GUCAS-VU Joint Lab for Social Computing and E-Health Research
Hebei University of Engineering, China
Nanjing University of Finance and Economics, China
National Natural Science Foundation of China
Victoria University, Australia
National Natural Science Foundation of China

Table of Contents

Keynotes Speech

Telehealth Strategies and Information Technology Transform Patient
Care within the U.S. Department of Veterans Affairs 1
  Leonard Goldschmidt

From Clinical Data to Knowledge Mining for Decision Making within
Hospitals 3
  Michael Steyn

Session 1

Building Socioemotional Environments in Metaverses for Virtual Teams
in Healthcare: A Conceptual Exploration........................... 4
  Xiaodan Yu, Dawn Owens, and Deepak Khazanchi

Integrating Healthcare-Related Information Using the Entity-Attribute-
Value Storage Model 13
  Dortje Löper, Meike Klettke, Ilvio Bruder, and Andreas Heuer

Median Polish with Power Transformations as an Alternative for the
Analysis of Contingency Tables with Patient Data.................. 25
  Frank Klawonn, Katja Crull, Akiko Kukita, and Frank Pessler

An Integrated Approach for Healthcare Planning over Multi-dimensional
Data Using Long-Term Prediction................................ 36
  Rui Henriques and Cláudia Antunes

A Novel Automated Recognition System Based on Medical Machining
CAD Models 49
  Hao Lan Zhang, Weitao Jiang, Huiqin Wu, and Libing Shu

Industry Perspective

Challenges and Opportunities for Health Information Systems
Research.. 60
  David Hansen

E-health in Australia – A General Practitioner's Perspective........... 61
  Stanley Chiang

Medical Devices: Panel Discussion................................. 62
  Terry Young

Session 2

Color Image Sharing Method Based on Lagrange's Interpolating
Polynomial   63
    Guiqiang Chen, Jianjun Liu, and Liqin Wang

Automation in Cytomics: A Modern RDBMS Based Platform for
Image Analysis and Management in High-Throughput Screening
Experiments   76
    E. Larios, Y. Zhang, K. Yan, Z. Di, S. LeDévédec,
    F. Groffen, and F.J. Verbeek

MRF Reconstruction of Retinal Images for the Optic Disc
Segmentation   88
    Ana Salazar-Gonzalez, Yongmin Li, and Djibril Kaba

Normalized Cut Segmentation of Thyroid Tumor Image Based on
Fractional Derivatives   100
    Jie Zhao, Li Zhang, Wei Zheng, Hua Tian, Dong-mei Hao, and
    Song-hong Wu

Cellular Neural Networks for Gold Immunochromatographic Strip
Image Segmentation   110
    Nianyin Zeng, Zidong Wang, Yurong Li, and Min Du

Session 3

A New Classification Method for Human Gene Splice Site Prediction . . .   121
    Dan Wei, Weiwei Zhuang, Qingshan Jiang, and Yanjie Wei

An Association Rule Analysis Framework for Complex Physiological
and Genetic Data   131
    Jing He, Yanchun Zhang, Guangyan Huang, Yefei Xin,
    Xiaohui Liu, Hao Lan Zhang, Stanley Chiang, and Hailun Zhang

Analysis of Nursery School Observations for Understanding Children's
Behavior   143
    Jien Kato and Yu Wang

Session 4

Epidemic Outbreak and Spread Detection System Based on Twitter
Data   152
    Xiang Ji, Soon Ae Chun, and James Geller

A Lightweight Approach for Extracting Disease-Symptom Relation
with MetaMap toward Automated Generation of Disease Knowledge
Base   164
    Takashi Okumura and Yuka Tateisi

Novel Hybrid Feature Selection Algorithms for Diagnosing
Erythemato-Squamous Diseases   173
    *Juanying Xie, Jinhu Lei, Weixin Xie, Xinbo Gao, Yong Shi, and
    Xiaohui Liu*

Author Index   187

Telehealth Strategies and Information Technology Transform Patient Care within the U.S. Department of Veterans Affairs

Leonard Goldschmidt

Ophthalmology Lead, VA Diabetic Teleretinal Screening Program
United States Department of Veterans Affairs (VA)
Palo Alto Health Care System
Palo Alto, California 94304
Leonard.Goldschmidt2@med.va.gov

For more than a decade, the U.S. Department of Veterans Affairs (VA) has pursued two linked strategies for the use of information technology (IT) in improving clinical health outcomes among the more than six million active patients under its care. The first strategy, implementation of computerized patient records (CPRS), was largely complete from 1999 onwards at the VA's 173 hospitals and more than 1000 community based outpatient clinics served by the organization in the United States. Many modifications have occurred since then, under the Veterans Health Information Systems and Technology Architecture (VistA), under which CPRS runs. The second major strategic program, taking advantage of CPRS but with its own advantages, has been the use of teleheath technologies. These are used to leverage medical specialty care and overcome the large geographic distances inherent in a health care system serving a widely dispersed population.

Within the past several years, these strategies have converged to form a major opportunity to serve our patients with improved organizational efficiency, enhanced patient safety, and desirable health care outcomes. "They've (VA) adopted a culture of patient safety and quality that is pervasive. The centerpiece of that culture is VistA, the VA's much praised electronic medical-records system[1]." Three major initiatives, in different stages of maturity, form the basis of telehealth within our organization. These include, Clinical Video Telehealth, Home Telehealth, and Store and Forward Telehealth. Each of these entities is supported by appropriate staffing involving training, administration, and supervision of clinical responsibility.

Clinical Video Telehealth encompasses dozens of medical and mental health diagnoses. Sessions typically occur over high bandwidth videoconferencing units, often connecting patients in remote community-based clinics with specialists in distant tertiary care centers. Using this modality means that the patient can see a specialist without the cost and inconvenience of long distance travel. Medications can be instituted or changed, and supplementary assessments performed using remote digital stethoscopes, ophthalmoscopes and other digitally supported devices. The computerized patient record is available, and notes and appropriate medical orders, e.g.,

---

[1] Business Week, July 17, 2006.

J. He et al. (Eds.): HIS 2012, LNCS 7231, pp. 1–2, 2012.
© Springer-Verlag Berlin Heidelberg 2012

medications, are entered with each visit. Over 200,000 of these encounters were performed throughout the health care system in 2011.

Home Telehealth springs from the realization that for many patients, serious illness necessitating urgent and emergency visits are days, weeks, and perhaps months in the making. Thus, by using a range of IT devices, many with interface to CPRS, data can be sent from the patient's home to a nurse or trained triage personnel who may evaluate the data and intervene with phone calls and home visits prior to devastating, preventable, and costly complications being noted in an emergency or intensive care setting. Digital peripherals using RS232 ports in the messaging devices include blood pressure, stethoscope, and even coagulation status assessment devices, among others. Diseases being treated in this manner include diabetes, heart failure, chronic pulmonary disease, hypertension, as well as several mental illnesses. Questions answered by the patient on home messaging devices are incorporated into algorithms programmed to assess a deteriorating clinical condition. These responses may be viewed on secure web sites by clinical personnel and a care coordination health plan formulated. Over 66,000 patients were treated in this manner in our system in 2011.

The final modality for telehealth in our health care system is store and forward telehealth, specifically for screening of diabetic retinopathy and for increased patient access to care using teledermatology. In place since 2006, the VA's diabetic screening program is among the largest in the world, approaching a million patients screened since the initiation of the program. The program is established in primary care medical clinics, as well as in eye clinics, to screen diabetic patients for this most common cause of preventable blindness. Commercial digital retinal cameras have a graphical interface to the VA computerized patient record, and images become part of the individual patient's health information. Retinal images are interpreted remotely, and often regionally, by trained eye professionals, with quality control measures incorporated as part of the training process for both imagers and readers. Over 171,000 studies were acquired in 2011.

The intersection of telehealth with a computerized patient record enables a variety of associated software tools to assume great importance. These tools include nascent phone applications for health, digital radiology acquisition and retrieval, medical decision support, online ordering of medications and instructions, patient education, medical library and drug information for the clinician, a clinical image archive supporting more than 65 different image file formats, and much more. This rich software architecture enables a work culture that emphasizes improving objective clinical outcome measures for many health conditions, as well as patient well-being. It is the marriage of an information technology and healthcare system that is absolutely necessary if health care is to be associated with making people more healthy, rather than simply treating their illnesses. In the future of our organization, these technology tools or mobile apps will be seen as means to an end, maintaining health in our veteran population, rather than programs with a life of their own. In the words of our leadership, "when fully implemented, telehealth will just be the way in which health care is provided. It will be nothing special, nor require a particular description[2].

Opinions expressed in this paper are not necessarily those of the Department of Veterans Affairs.

---

[2] http://www.telehealth.va.gov

From Clinical Data to Knowledge Mining for Decision Making within Hospitals

(Keynote Speech)

Michael Steyn

What are we doing and why? Why should we integrate our expertise and professions – what is the value of us forming teams – just because we can, does not mean we should? There has to be a common goal, a reason for our endeavors. Most importantly this must translate into change – a better outcome for our patients, our communities and ourselves.

So we embark on a journey examining 3 linked pathways:

1. The doctor patient interaction and our care for a community – the clinical approach to solving issues for an individual, the development of answers for a community and our use of pattern recognition, memory and gambling.
2. The building and management of knowledge – the crucial linkage of data into information, with progression to knowledge and the aim of achieving wisdom.
3. The role of information technology in clinical medicine (using anaesthesia as an example) – how it changed, how it is changing with the impact of a State-wide Automatic Anaesthesia Record (WinChart, Medtel) and most importantly the future with research into real time data integration, pattern recognition and decision support.

The theme of this trip is "what are we doing" and "why are we doing" but remember the target - what difference are we making or more importantly should we make! And the correct destination is…

J. He et al. (Eds.): HIS 2012, LNCS 7231, p. 3, 2012.
© Springer-Verlag Berlin Heidelberg 2012

Building Socioemotional Environments in Metaverses for Virtual Teams in Healthcare: A Conceptual Exploration

Xiaodan Yu[1,*], Dawn Owens[2], and Deepak Khazanchi[2]

[1] College of Information Science and Technology, University of Nebraska at Omaha, U.S.A.
Research Center on Fictitious Economy and Data Science, CAS,Beijing 100190, China
{xyu}@mail.unomaha.edu
[2] College of Information Science and Technology, University of Nebraska at Omaha, U.S.A.
{dmowens,khazanchi}@mail.unomaha.edu

Abstract. Metaverses are 3-dimentional (3D) virtual environments that allow people to interact with each other through software agents without physical limitations. There is great interest in the use of Metaverses for health and medical education. This paper examines the application of metaverses for supporting effective collaboration and knowledge sharing in virtual teams. Virtual teams have been used in health/medical area, such as home healthcare. However, the management of virtual teams is challenging. This study proposes that metaverses have the potential to provide socioemotional environments where individuals socially interact with others. Such socioemotional environments have the potential to facilitate effective collaboration and knowledge sharing in virtual teams. Building on previous research, we developed a conceptual model for understanding how metaverses enable the development of social-emotional environments in virtual teams.

Keywords: Metaverse, Virtual teams, Socioemotional environment, Collaboration.

1 Introduction

Virtual teams (VTs) consist of geographically dispersed individuals who work interdependently toward a common goal [1]. Virtual teams have been used in health/medical area, such as home healthcare [2]. Numerous information and communication technologies (ICTs), such as email, groupware, instant online communication tools, support the needs of virtual teams in terms of communication, coordination and control [3]. For example, many international virtual teams adopt common net-based workspaces to share and create objects of work among participants [4]. The interdisciplinary nature of e-health has brought a lot of attention from researchers in medical science, computer science [24-27], information systems, and management science [28-36].

One example of newer ICT is the metaverse. A metaverse is an immersive 3D space where people can interact with each other through avatars and software agents.

J. He et al. (Eds.): HIS 2012, LNCS 7231, pp. 4–12, 2012.

Thanks to their unique capabilities, metaverses have gained attention from both practitioners and academics. Sun is building a virtual world for its employees with the purpose of recreating a real-life interaction in an office [5]; IBM, with approximately 3,200 engineers and scientists at eight labs in six countries, also started to "open the virtual doors" to achieve collaborative innovations. Figure 1 shows a Second Life conference room where Oracle gives orientation to its newly acquired employees. In addition to business applications, metaverses have also been used in Universities, hospitals, and government. Imperial College London has created a "virtual hospital" inside Second Life (Fig. 2.)

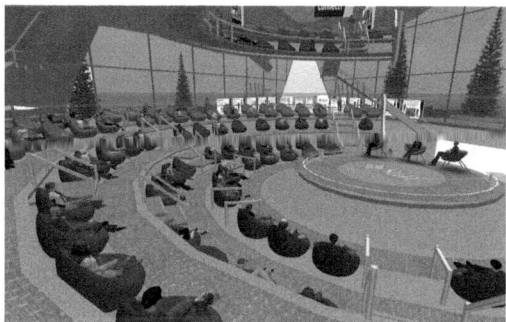

Fig. 1. Oracle holding a conference using Second Life
(http://blogs.oracle.com/vw/entry/a_look_back_at_the)

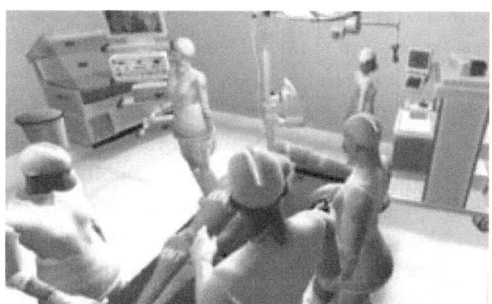

Fig. 2. Medical training in second life
(http://www.vizworld.com/2009/07/can-training-in-second-life-teach-doctors-to-save-real-lives/)

Why does metaverse technology draw so much attention by business and academics? Research has suggested that metaverse technology, with its unique capabilities, has greater potential for rich and engaging collaboration than the other ICT tools [6, 7]. Metaverse technology not only provides instrumental features—task-specific features--, but also has the capabilities for creating a socioemotional environment. Though other ICT tools, such as email, telephone, and video-conferencing, aim at mimicking face-to-face communication, none of them provides a common environment for individuals to visually interact as they virtually collaborate. Within such a common environment, there is the potential for individuals in virtual teams to build trust, shared understanding and thus experience enhanced team outcomes [8]. Research has established that more effective communication and team outcomes are found in a socioemotional, or social richness, environment [9].

Thus, the purpose of this paper is to enhance our understanding about the development of a socioemotional environment using metaverse technology. Specifically, our goal is to understand how metaverses can support socioemotional environment building. We address this goal in the form of a conceptual model, which builds on Davis et al.'s conceptual model for metaverse research [3].

2   Metaverses

Metaverses are immersive three-dimensional virtual worlds (VWs) in which people interact as avatars with each other and with software agents, using the metaphor of the real world but without its physical limitations [6]. One of examples of a metaverse is Second Life. Empirical research has found that VTs experience more effective collaboration in the context of metaverses than other ICT tools [10, 11]. One stream of research in metaverse technology has taken a technology-centric perspective to studying the use of metaverses in VTs. This stream of research is based on media-richness theory and suggests that metaverses permit effective collaboration because of its rich media characteristics. Compared to other ICT tools, such as video-conferencing, metaverses are able to transmit non-verbal cues as facial expression and gaze, which allows turn-taking.   This permits individuals to render their appearances and to change their position in the environment [12].

A second stream of research in studying the effective use of metaverses takes a behavioral perspective by studying the psychological or social consequences associated with the use of metaverses. From the behavioral perspective, metaverses are described as an immersive and highly interactive environment [13] where individuals experience high degrees of social presence, co-presence, and trust [6, 14].

Davis et al. [6] took a socio-technical perspective which integrates the above two approaches to examine the metaverses. They suggest that effective use of metaverses is a function both of the technology capabilities inherent in metaverses and of the ongoing social interaction by individuals. They proposed a conceptual model to account for the dynamic capabilities and behaviors in metaverses environment. Consistent with the adaptive structuration theory, they view the use of technologies is an adaptive process during which users make modifications regarding what capabilities to use and how to use the capabilities. In their model, Davis et al. [6] identified five components, namely metaverse, people/avatars, metaverse technology capabilities, behaviors, and outcomes. Metaverses are the immersive virtual environment where people interact with others as avatars. People/avatars refer to the digital representation of people created by individuals. Metaverse technology capabilities are categorized into four areas, communication, rendering, interaction, and team process tools. Behaviors include any actions executed by people as they communicate and interact with others in metaverses. Outcomes are measures chosen to evaluate the effectiveness of virtual teams.

The model [6] is an iterative model to account for the complex interplay among these five components. In this paper we extend on this conceptual model by including the socioemotional component to account for the use of metaverses in building social richness environments.

3   Conceptual Model Development

Extending the conceptual model proposed by Davis et al. [6], we include another component, referred to as socioemotional environment, as is shown in Figure 3, to account for the psychological consequences that may affect and be affected by meta-verse technology capabilities.

The notion of "socioemotional" can be traced back in the Bales' (1950) equilibrium model: a group continuously divides its attention between instrumental (task-related) needs and expressive (socioemotional). Socioemotional refers to an environment that is social richness. Socioemtional environment emphasizes the capabilities of ICT in providing a social environment rather than merely a work platform to accomplish particular tasks [15]. Research has suggested that a socialemotional environment is more effective in supporting communication and task performance [15]. Though there are many constructs in examining the socioemotional environment, we are par-ticularly interested in those that have the greatest likelihood to be impacted by tech-nology as well as those that impact outcomes. Specifically, we are interested in these two constructs of social presence, and social verification. Thus we define socioemo-tional environment as *a technology mediated environment, where people communi-cate with others and perceive strong sense of presence and social interactions with others.*

Consistent with Davis et al.'s perspective, we view the process of building a so-cioemotional environment in the context of metaverse as a dynamic and adaptive process. To put it another way, the use of metaverses by people emerges from the on-going interactions between metaverses and people. Virtual team members may ex-perience different degrees of socioemotional environment by following different paths or patterns of behaviors in metaverses.

While prior design of ICT focuses on the features of supporting task-driven activi-ties, current trends suggest the importance of developing the socioemotional aspects of support [14, 16]. Considering the scope of this paper, that means IT needs to be designed to enhance participants' feeling of social presence and social verification.

Social presence has been widely used in communication research in theorizing numerous ICTs. Further, it has become one of the most important criteria in designing and assessing media products. Similar concepts used to refer to social presence are telepresence [17-19], virtual presence [17], and mediated presence [9]. Considering the purpose of this paper, we chose to use social presence, defined as "a psychological state in which virtual (para-authentic or artificial) objects are experienced as actual objects in either sensory or nonsensory ways" [20].

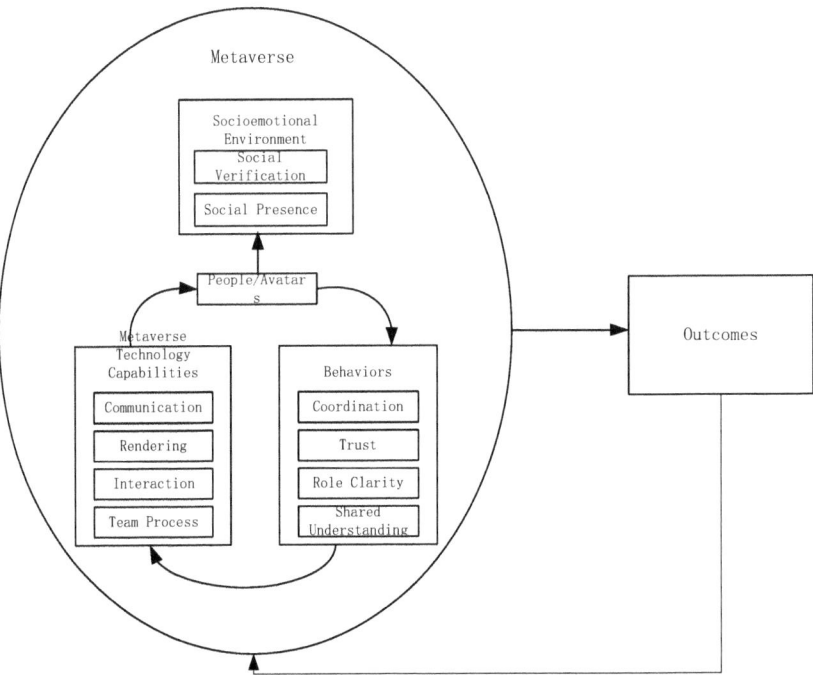

Fig. 3. Model for Building a Socioemotional Environment Using Metaverse Technology Capabilities [adapted from [6]]

Further, Lee [20] suggests that social presence is related to individual's virtual experience which consists of three components--physical experience, social experience, and individual experience. Physical experience occurs when individuals interact with physical artifacts through ICTs or when individuals interact with physical artifacts created by ICTs. Social experience is about the social actors. When individuals interact through ICT or individuals interact with ICT-enabled social actors, individuals are having virtual social experience. People experience refers to experience when individuals' own selves are constructed by technology.

After examining social presence and its relating three components of virtual experience, we anticipate that metaverses have the potential for enhanced social presence in several areas. First, metaverses provide a common environment, which is essential for developing antecedents to social presence, such as shared attention, common ground building, situated communication, and awareness [21]. The capability to create a shared space provides virtual team members a feeling of "elsewhere", rather than of "here and there" [14, 22]. Second, metaverses' rendering capability permits individuals to freely show their personalities and preferences through manipulating their avatars. The flexibility of changing the appearances and the positions enhances individual's perception of being presence. Based upon the discussion, we propose:

> *Proposition 1: Metaverse technologies provide capabilities for shared environment and rendering, the interplay and on-going use of these capabilities affect people/avatars' sense of social presence.*

Whereas social presence focuses on describing individual's psychological state about own self, social verification is a concept relating to individual's perceptions about his/her relationship with others. Consistent with Blascovich [23], we define social verification as "the extent to which participants in virtual groups experience interactions with virtual others in ways that verify that they are engaging in semantically meaningful communication with virtual others thereby experiencing shared reality". This definition about social verification suggests that individuals will experience high degree of social verification if he/she is engaging or engaged meaningful communication with others in a shared environment. Thus, effective communication and shared environment are two important antecedents to developing social verification.

Metaverses are designed to mimic the face-to-face interactions without physical limitations. For example, the use of positioning allows virtual team members to represent themselves in a manner highly reminiscent of face-to-face conversations. In an empirical study of metaverses for virtual teams, Owen et al. [8] found that with interaction capabilities such as mobility, interactivity, and immediacy of artifacts, virtual team members are seen less challenge in terms of coordination and communication by visually show their skills. Besides, the synchronous nature of metaverse technology ensures that all members share the progress of the task in a timely manner. Thus, we propose:

> *Proposition 2: Metaverse technologies provide capabilities for communication, team process and interaction, the interplay and on-going use of these capabilities affect people/avatars' sense of social verification.*

Based upon the above discussion about social presence and social verification, we propose:

> *Proposition 3: Metaverse technologies provide capabilities for shared environment, communication, team process and interaction, the interplay and on-going use of these capabilities affect people/avatars' sense of being in a socioemotional environment.*

4　Conclusion

Our purpose is to examine how metaverses can be used to build a socioemotional environment. Our conceptual model and propositions suggest a new way of exploring the use of metaverses for effective virtual team collaborations. Metaverses are different from traditional collaboration technologies. With unique capabilities, metaverses have great potential in supporting a socioemotional environment where effective collaboration and knowledge sharing can be achieved. The conceptual model and propositions enhance our understanding about the potential of using metaverses for supporting collaboration and knowledge sharing in virtual teams in health/medical application. Future research should empirically evaluate the model in order to gain a more in-depth understanding about the use of metaverses for building socioemotional environments.

References

1. Powell, A., Piccoli, G., Ives, B.: Virtual teams: A review of current literature and directions for future research. Database for Advances in Information Systems 35(1), 6–36 (2004)
2. Pitsillides, A., et al.: DITIS: Virtual collaborative teams for home healthcare. Journal of Mobile Multimedia 2(1) (2006)
3. Khazanchi, D., Zigurs, I.: Patterns for effective management of virtual projects: Theory and evidence. International Journal of Electronic Collaboration 2(3), 25–49 (2006)
4. Majchrzak, A., et al.: Technology adaptation: The case of a computer supported inter-organizational virtual team. MIS Quarterly 24(4), 569–600 (2000)
5. Brodkin, J.: Sun building collaborative, virtual world (2007)
6. Davis, A., et al.: Avatars, people, and metaverses: Foundations for research in metaverses. Journal of the Association for Information Systems 10(2), 99–117 (2009)
7. Bainbridge, W.S.: The scientific research potential of virtual worlds. Science 317, 472–476 (2007)
8. Owens, D., et al.: An empirical investigation of virtual world projects and metaverse technology capabilities. The DATA BASE for Advances in Information Systems 42(1), 74–101 (2011)
9. Biocca, F., Harms, C., Burgoon, J.: Criteria and scope conditions for a theory and measure of social presence. In: Presence 2001, 4th Annual International Workshop, Philadelphia, PA (2001)
10. Schroeder, R., Heldal, I., Tromp, J.: The usability of collaborative virtual environments and methods for the analysis of interaction. Presence 16(5), 655–667 (2006)
11. Sempsey, J.J., Johnston, D.A.: The psychological dynamics and social climate of text-based virtual reality. Journal of Virtual Environments 5(1) (2000)
12. Anderson, A., Dossick, C.S., Iorio, J.: Avatars, Text, and Miscommunication: The Impact of Communication Richness on Global Virtual Team Collaboration. Working Paper (2011)
13. Magnenat-Thalmann, N., Kim, H., Egges, A., Garchery, S.: Believability and Interaction in Virtual Worlds. In: Proceedings of the 11th International Multimedia Modelling Conference, Melbourne, Australia (2005)
14. Bente, G., et al.: Avatar-mediated networking: Increasing social presence and interpersonal trust in net-based collaborations. Human Communication Research 34(2), 287–318 (2008)
15. Redfern, S., Naughton, N.: Collaborative virtual environments to support communication and community in internet-based distance education. Journal of Information Technology Education 1(3) (2002)
16. Tanis, M., Postmes, T.: Social cues and impression formation in CMC. Journal of Communication 53, 676–693 (2003)

17. Sheridan, T.B.: Musings on telepresence and virtual presence. Presence: Teleoperators and Virtual Environments 1, 120–126 (1992)
18. Slater, M., Usoh, M.: Representations systems, perceptual position, and presence in immersive virtual environments. Presence: Teleoperators and Virtual Environments 2, 221–233 (1993)
19. Rheingold, H.: Virtual reality. Summit Books, New York (1991)
20. Lee, K.M.: Presence, Explicated. Communication Theory 14(1), 27–50 (2004)
21. Whittaker, S.: Theories and methods in mediated communciation. In: Graesser, M.G.A., Goldman, S. (eds.) The Hand Book of Discourse Processes, pp. 243–286. Lawrence Erlbaum Associates, Mahwah (2002)
22. Foster, D., Meech, J.: The social dimensions of virtual reality. In: Carr, K., England, R. (eds.) Simulated and Virtual Realities: Elements of Perception. Taylor and Francis, London (1995)
23. Blascovich, J.: A theoretical model of social influence for increasing the utility of collaborative virtual environments. In: Proceedings of the 4th International Conference on Collaborative Virtual Environments 2002, Bonn, Germany. ACM, New York (2002)
24. Shi, Y., Zhang, X., Wan, J., Kou, G., Peng, Y., Guo, Y.: Comparison study of two kernel-based learning algorithms for predicting the distance range between antibody interface residues and antigen surface. International Journal of Computer Mathematics 84, 690–707 (2007)
25. Shi, Y., Zhang, X., Wan, J., Wang, Y., Ying, W., Cao, Z., Guo, Y.: Predicting the Distance between Antibody's Interface Residue And Antigen To Recognize Antigen Types By Support Vector Machine. Neural Computing & Applications 16, 481–490 (2007)
26. Zheng, J., Zhuang, W., Yan, N., Kou, G., Erichsen, D., McNally, C., Peng, H., Cheloha, A., Shi, C., Shi, Y.: Classification of HIV-1 Mediated Neuronal Dendritic and Synaptic Damage Using Multiple Criteria Linear Programming. Neuroinformatics 2, 303–326 (2004)
27. Chen, Z.Y., Li, J.P., Wei, L.W.: A multiple kernel support vector machine scheme for feature selection and rule extraction from gene expression data of cancer tissue. Artificial Intelligence in Medicine 41(2), 161–175 (2007)
28. Kou, G., Peng, Y., Chen, Z., Shi, Y.: Multiple criteria mathematical programming for multi-class classification and application in network intrusion detection. Information Sciences 179(4), 371–381 (2009)
29. Shi, Y., Tian, Y., Chen, X., Zhang, P.: Regularized Multiple Criteria Linear Programs for Classification. Science in China Series F: Information Sciences 52, 1812–1820 (2009)
30. Peng, Y., Kou, G., Shi, Y., Chen, Z.: A Descriptive Framework for the Field of Data Mining and Knowledge Discovery. International Journal of Information Technology and Decision Making 7(4), 639–682 (2008)
31. Peng, Y., Kou, G., Shi, Y., Chen, Z.: A Multi-Criteria Convex Quadratic Programming Model for Credit Data Analysis. Decision Support Systems 44, 1016–1030 (2008)
32. Cheng, S., Dai, R., Xu, W., Shi, Y.: Research on Data Mining and Knowledge Management and Its Applications in China's Economic Development: Significance and Trend. International Journal of Information Technology and Decision Making 5(4), 585–596 (2006)
33. Shi, Y., Peng, Y., Kou, G., Chen, Z.: Classifying Credit Card Accounts for Business Intelligence and Decision Making: A Multiple-Criteria Quadratic Programming Approach. International Journal of Information Technology and Decision Making 4, 581–600 (2005)

34. Kou, G., Peng, Y., Shi, Y., Wise, M., Xu, W.: Discovering Credit Cardholders' Behavior by Multiple Criteria Linear Programming. Annals of Operations Research 135, 261–274 (2005)
35. He, J., Liu, X., Shi, Y., Xu, W., Yan, N.: Classifications of Credit Cardholder Behavior by using Fuzzy Linear Programming. International Journal of Information Technology and Decision Making 3, 633–650 (2004)
36. Zheng, J., Zhuang, W., Yan, N., Kou, G., Erichsen, D., McNally, C., Peng, H., Cheloha, A., Shi, C., Shi, Y.: Classification of HIV-1 Mediated Neuronal Dendritic and Synaptic Damage Using Multiple Criteria Linear Programming. Neuroinformatics 2, 303–326 (2004)

Integrating Healthcare-Related Information Using the Entity-Attribute-Value Storage Model

Dortje Löper, Meike Klettke, Ilvio Bruder, and Andreas Heuer

Database Research Group
University of Rostock, 18051 Rostock, Germany
{dortje.loeper,meike.klettke,ilvio.bruder,andreas.heuer}@uni-rostock.de

Abstract. For an optimal care of patients in home healthcare, it is essential to exchange healthcare-related information with other stakeholders. Unfortunately, paper-based documentation procedures as well as the heterogeneity between information systems inhibit a well-regulated communication. Therefore, a digital patient care record is introduced to establish the foundation for integrating healthcare-related information. To overcome the heterogeneity, standards for health information exchange such as HL7 CDA are used. This paper proposes a generic storage structure based on the entity-attribute-value (EAV) model for the patient care record. This approach offers flexibility concerning different standard types and the evolution in healthcare knowledge and processes. It also allows for highly sparsed data to be stored in a compact way.

The underlying database structure is presented, the import process for extracting incoming reports is described and the export process for generating new outgoing standardized reports is briefly illustrated. First performance tests regarding the query response time are also given.

1 Introduction

In home healthcare, manual paperwork is still in use in several scenarios. Especially in Germany, a paper-based documentation of the fulfilled care activities including some special reports is required to reside in the patient's home and needs to be synchronized with the data in the care information system regularly. Additionally, the information is usually exchanged with other stakeholders via paper-based reports, too, and sometimes even needs to be explicitly requested.

Transferring information from paper to a digital format always implies additional time and effort. Furthermore, this manual work is error-prone and hence might be harmful for the patient's healthcare. In addition to that, new information can only be accessed after a certain delay.

Our vision is to provide the home healthcare personnel with a mobile device to support the documentation process as stated by Umblia et al. [16] and to replace the paper-based patient care record by a digital one at the patient's home. Hence, the care information system, the mobile device and the digital care record can synchronize their patient's information automatically. Moreover, the patient care record can be used for integrating other stakeholder's information. In order

J. He et al. (Eds.): HIS 2012, LNCS 7231, pp. 13–24, 2012.

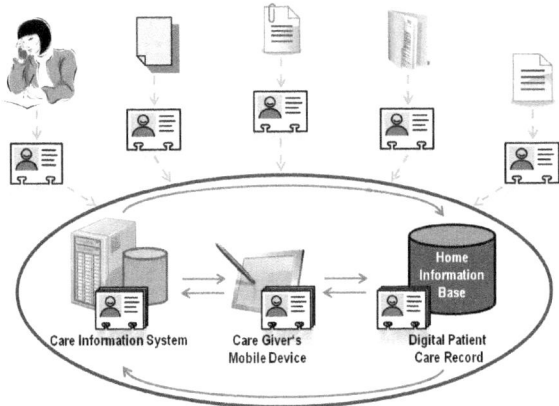

Fig. 1. Vision of Information Integration in Home Healthcare

to bypass the heterogeneity of the different stakeholder's information systems, standardized healthcare reports are expected to be used for the exchange of data. This vision is shown in figure 1.

An open issue is the storage structure of the digital care record. In order to include a wide variety of different information and different standards, a generic approach is necessary. Additionally, the knowledge as well as the processes are continuously developed both in the medical and in the healthcare area. Therefore, the approach should be flexible enough to handle this evolution. This paper deals with the development of a storage structure based on the entity-attribute-value model and introduces the import and export processes for this structure.

The remainder of this article is structured as follows: Section 2 provides an overview of the state of the art on integrating healthcare information and briefly describes some common healthcare standards. The following section 3 introduces the entity-attribute-value model and suggests a suitable storage structure. Moreover, the import and export processes as well as data privacy in this sensitive domain are discussed. Results of a general performance evaluation are presented in section 4. Finally, section 5 concludes with a summary and an outlook.

2   Information Integration in the Home Care Scenario

Supplying care givers with the right information in the right place at the right time is essential in home healthcare. Conflicts resulting from fragmented information can become a threat to a patient's safety [8]. Moreover, this information should be provided automatically avoiding additional time and effort. In this article, an approach for a central data management is introduced. But first, an overview of existing technologies in the healthcare domain is given.

2.1   Related Work on Information Integration in Healthcare

Lenz et al. [11,12] examine the general problem context of information integration in (mainly German) healthcare networks. They describe the information systems in these networks as being highly heterogeneous and having interfaces which lack flexibility. Along with a classification of current communication standards for interoperability in healthcare, they also present a list of requirements for integrating healthcare-related information. In order to achieve more interoperability, an incremental approach is proposed and generic models are predicted to be the basis for IT systems.

Sunyaev et al. use a multi agent architecture for integrating health information [15]. Therein, the basic medical treatment process is mapped to agent-based technology. The key feature of the system is an active document which virtually collects requested information about one patient. However, mobile agents introduce safety hazards, which is a major drawback of this approach.

The treatment process can also be mapped to a document-based workflow [14]. While traversing the workflow elements, information units are collected from engaged institutions. Together, these information units form a resulting document representing the whole treatment process information. Both, this and the preceding approach focus on the treatment process and the composition of corresponding information. On the other hand, the digital patient record that will be presented in the article at hand expects self-contained reports.

While the two previous approaches focus on the treatment process, Haegglund et al. aim at generally integrating healthcare information from different sources [9]. Data is exported from the information system, mapped to an ideal XML schema and stored in a mediator database. The stakeholders access this database via mobile applications. However, due to a restricted application context, there are only three fixed data sources. A new information systems can't be added automatically, a new mapping to the ideal XML format must be provided.

The last approach presented herein deals with a middleware platform to exchange messages between different healthcare institutions [1]. Building on different types of message standards and protocols, a client-server-architecture is implemented together with an enterprise service bus in order to separate the data transmission from the data processing. While this approach focuses on the transfer of data, the digital patient care record could be seen as one client in the scenario.

2.2   Standards for Health Information Communication

Standards are being developed in different areas in order to have a common concept on syntax and semantics of certain data and to ensure interoperability. In the envisioned home healthcare scenario, information from other stakeholders are expected to be received in form of standardized reports. Examples for standards which determine the structural content comprise the HL7 Clinical Document Architecture (CDA) and the CEN ENV 13606 Electronic Healthcare Record Communication (EHRcom).

Different stakeholders are interested in different parts of the overall healthcare information and deliver different information units. These may also be provided in different standards or different templates of standards. For example, the HL7 family specifies the CDA as a generic base document. With the help of implementation guidelines and templates, this generic structure can be restricted to a well-specified subarea. Examples of German implementation guides are the eArztbrief [7], a consultation note for communicating information from one physician to another one, and the ePflegebericht[5] to transmit healthcare information, e.g. from a home healthcare giver to a stationary one.

Furthermore, terminologies and classifications are used to specify uniform concepts and processes within the medical and healthcare domain. In the healthcare domain, the International Classification of Nursing Practice (ICNP) which has been developed by the International Council of Nurses (ICN) and the nursing terminology developed by the NANDA-I are examples for such classifications.

2.3 The Digital Patient Care Record as the Main Healthcare Information Storage

The digital patient care record serves as an integration center for all healthcare information that is delivered by standardized reports from other stakeholders. At the same time, it is supposed to be the source for generating new standardized reports to be sent to other care participants. Hence, it represents the main home healthcare information storage for a patient.

Regarding one single patient, healthcare as well as medical data is highly sparsed. A storage structure must be able to handle that efficiently. Additionally, it should fulfill the following requirements:

- *Flexibility*: in order to include reports that are based on different standards or standard templates
- *Stability concerning model updates*: to allow for incorporating new versions of standards or complete new standards in the future
- *Versioning*: to reproduce changes of data
- *Restorability*: the original reports have to be available
- *Traceability*: it is necessary to establish the provenience for each data
- *Extensibility*: in order to adapt to the constantly evolving knowledge and processes in healthcare

In the following, the entity-attribute-value model will be presented as a basis for a generic storage structure for the digital patient care record.

3 The Entity-Attribute-Value Model

The entity-attribute-value model offers a generic approach for storing different kinds of information by not only storing the actual values but also reflecting the structure of the information as values in the database. The main advantage is the higher degree of flexibility concerning structural differences in the incoming information.

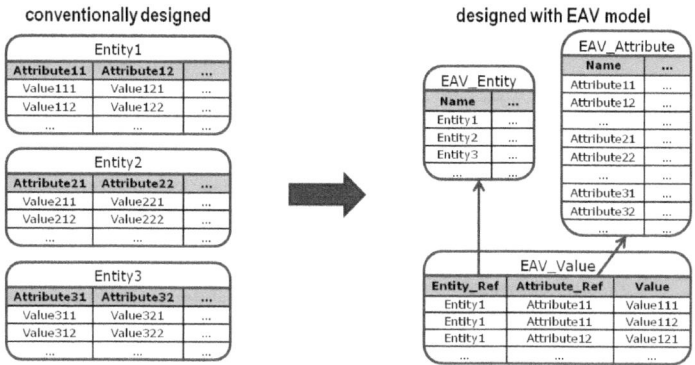

Fig. 2. The basic Concept of Entity-Attribute-Value Modeling

3.1   The Main Concept of the Entity-Attribute-Value Model

The entity-attribute-value model comprises three basic relations (as shown in figure 2): the actual data are stored in the relation *value* whereas the entities and the attributes are stored in the relations *entity* and *attribute*, respectively.

The EAV model has already been used in different domains. In the health-related areas it is used to store and manage highly sparsed patient data in a compact and efficient way [2,3,6,13]. The main advantages of the entity-attribute-value model are:

- *Compact storage handling*: Highly sparsed data are stored in a compact way.
- *Flexible and extensible model*: This model is highly flexible, because different types of data objects can be included, even if the underlying format is different. Also different types or implementations of standards can be supported.
- *Stability concerning model updates*: The model is also flexible regarding the evolution of data sources. New schema versions of XML-based standards or relational databases don't require any modification in the EAV structure or the already stored data. The same applies for adding new data sources.
- *Simple restoring capabilities*: No data transformation is required in order to store the incoming information, the entities, attributes and values remain the same. No data is lost. This is especially crucial in medical applications because of the patient's sensitive data.

These features mainly cover the requirements presented in section 2.3: The EAV-model is flexible, updateable, extensible and the information is recoverable. For achieving traceability, the value relation(s) can store a reference to the source document. Versioning can be achieved by extending the EAV model.

On the one hand, the generic storage structure is convenient regarding input operations and the storage of heterogeneous and highly-sparsed data. On the other hand, the query response time is adversely affected, especially with respect to attribute-centric queries [2]. For larger amounts of data this effect increases.

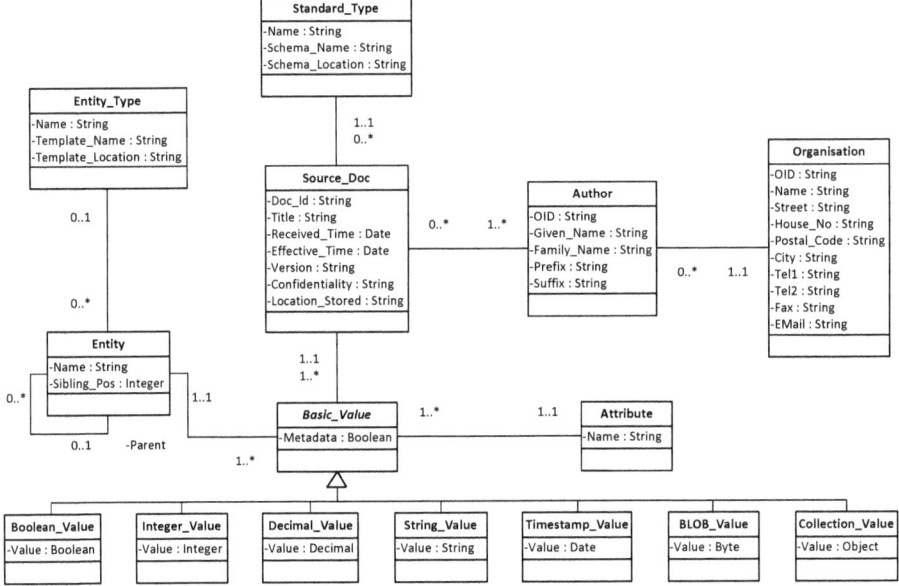

Fig. 3. Basic Class Model of the EAV Storage Structure

Thus, the entity-attribute-value model only pays off in certain applications which need flexibility. In many cases, the EAV model isn't used exclusively but along with a conventional database schema in order to combine the advantages of both formats for different classes of data [13].

In our scenario, the data volume is relatively small, because the ambulant care givers are responsible for one patient or a restricted number of patients only. Hence, the impact on performance is expected to be relatively low.

3.2 The Entity-Attribute-Value Concept as a Global Schema for Information Integration

The digital patient care record with the underlying EAV storage model provides the basis for integrating all care-relevant information. We extended the original EAV model by introducing separate value tables for different data types (similar to the suggestions in [4] and [13]).

We developed a storage structure based on the extended EAV model. Figure 3 represents the basic schema of our database storage structure. All data types that are enumerated in the ISO standard 21090 [10] can be stored in the model. For reflecting hierarchical structures (e.g. derived from XML documents), an attribute *Parent* was added in the entity relation. Moreover, an attribute *Sibling_Pos* refers to the position of an entity among its siblings.

Listing 1.1. Extract of a Health Record based on HL7 CDA

```
...
<entry typeCode="DRIV">
  <observation classCode="OBS" moodCode="EVN">
    <code code="29308-4" codeSystem="2.16.840.113883.6.1"/>
    <statusCode code= "completed"/>
    <effectiveTime> <low value="20090313"/> </effectiveTime>
    <value xsi:type="CD" code="A01.5" codeSystem="2.16.840.1.113883.6.236"
      codeSystemName="CCC" displayName="Physical Mobility Impairment">
      <originalText> <reference value="#diag-1"/> </originalText>
      <qualifier>
        <name code="8" codeSystem="2.16.840.1.113883.3.7.1"/>
        <value code="G" codeSystem="2.16.840.1.113883.3.7.1.8"
          displayName="confirmed diagnosis"/>
      </qualifier>
    </value>
  </observation>
</entry>
...
```

Due to the fact that, e.g. in HL7 CDA, many attributes can be used within a large number of entities, there is no direct connection between the attribute relation and the entity relation. A relationship between those tables would result in a repeated and redundant storage of the same attribute in the attribute table. The combination of entity and attribute is derived from the respective value relation instead.

Additionally, each value relation also holds foreign keys to some general information about the source document which are stored in metadata relations. These metadata comprise data about the source document including the author and possible document types and templates. Also, a boolean attribute *Metadata* refers to whether the data is extracted from the header part of the document (which usually contains metadata like physician's information as well as general information about the patient and the document) or from the body part of the document (containing the actual medical or healthcare information).

In the following, an example is presented which illustrates the mapping of a standardized document to the EAV storage structure. Listing 1.1 depicts a part of a standardized healthcare document as an instance of the German ePegebericht, which is based on HL7 CDA (the example is taken from [5]). Figure 4 displays how this document is mapped to the EAV storage structure. For simplification purposes, only those tables are shown which contain data from the example. Importantly, all the XML elements reside in the entity relation, and the XML attributes are stored in the attribute relation, respectively. The value relations contain the actual values along with references to the corresponding attribute, entity and source_doc entry.

3.3   Transformation Processes

In the previous sections, the integrated EAV format for storing medical and healthcare records was introduced. We initially assumed that incoming data and documents are available in different standards. Furthermore, reports and documents have to comply with different standards or different versions of standards, as well. Therefore, import and export processes have to be defined.

Entity				
Id	Name	Type	Parent	Sibling_Pos
5	entry	-	2	1
6	obeservation	-	5	1
7	code	-	6	1
8	statusCode	-	6	2
9	effectiveTime	-	6	3
10	value	-	6	4
11	originalText	-	10	1
12	qualifier	-	10	2
13	name	-	12	1
14	value	-	12	2
15	reference	-	11	1
16	low	-	9	1
...	...	...	...	...

Attribute	
Id	Name
1	code
2	codeSystem
3	ID
4	textField
5	typeCode
6	classCode
7	moodCode
8	value
9	Xsi:type
10	codeSystemName
11	displayName
...	...

String_Value					
Id	Source	Entity	Attribute	M.	Value
5	1	5	5	0	DRIV
6	1	6	6	0	OBS
7	1	6	7	0	EVN
8	1	8	1	0	Completed
9	1	16	8	0	20090313
10	1	10	9	0	CD
11	1	10	1	0	A01.5
12	1	10	2	0	2.16.840.1.113883.6.236
13	1	10	10	0	CCC
14	1	10	11	0	Physical Mobil. Impairment
15	1	15	8	0	#diag-1
16	1	13	1	0	8
17	1	13	2	0	2.16.840.1.113883.3.7.1
18	1	10	1	0	G
19	1	10	2	0	2.16.840.1.113883.3.7.1.8
20	1	10	11	0	Confirmed Diagnosis
...	...	...	...	...	...

Integer_Value					
Id	Source	Entity	Attribute	M.	Value
18	1	13	1	0	8
...	...	...	...	...	...

Fig. 4. Storing the above Example in the EAV Storage Structure

The import process is pretty straightforward. The subtasks that transform a document into the EAV model are shown in figure 5. This process can be completely automated, even for new database sources or new XML document formats. Usually, no support by the domain expert is needed. All necessary information can be derived from the source databases or source XML documents. Only in case of new data formats (for instance: hierarchical databases or Excel data sheets) the import transformation component has to be extended.

The EAV model stores the original data from the sources without any information loss. Compared to other integration scenarios, that is a significant advantage, because it ensures restorability of all integrated documents.

Exporting data from the EAV model is more complicated, though. We have to overcome the heterogeneities introduced by the different data sources. Figure 6 shows the subtasks for the export process. In most cases, newly generated reports only contain a fraction of the stored patient data. The selection of the data to be exported can be divided into two steps: The care giver gets a preselected list of data, e.g. which are shown on a mobile device, and then chooses the relevant data among this list manually.

The most complicated task within the export process is the *Transformation*. For this task, transformation rules are applied for the mapping of data, which are either prepared (available in the system for known data formats) or have to be extended by the domain expert for new and previously unknown data formats.

The next subtask is a test of *Completeness* where the system checks whether the generated documents are valid and contain all necessary data. Otherwise, for instance if not all personal data of a patient are contained in the document, then the data selection is repeated. This process is performed until a valid export document is generated.

If new databases, databases with evolved structure or documents which unknown XML schemas are integrated into the system, the transformation needs to be extended.

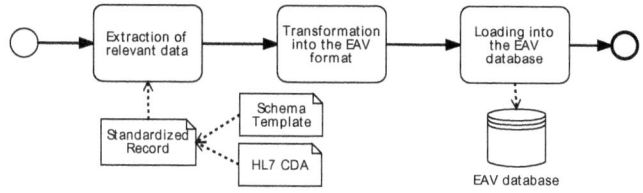

Fig. 5. Import Process: Mapping a Standardized Report to the EAV Storage Structure

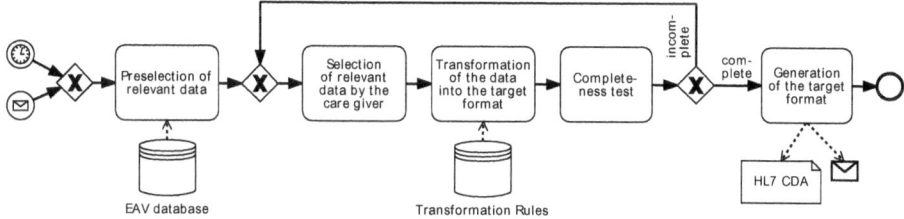

Fig. 6. Export Process: Generating a new Standardized Report

3.4   Data Security and Access Rights for the EAV Storage Solution

In our approach for home healthcare, sensitive data about a patient are collected and stored in a database. The protection of this sensitive medical data is necessary. The storage solution has to ensure that only authorized persons and user groups can change or access the data. Therefore individual rights for specific users or groups have to be set properly to allow access to well-specified portions of the data.

The EAV storage solution stores all values in the same relation. Because database management systems can specify access rights for users only on complete tables, the view concept of databases has to be applied. Views can be defined to select data from the original EAV database. Database systems allow to specify access rights for reading, adding, deleting and updating data for each view separately and subsequently for the corresponding fractions of data.

Hence, horizontal and vertical fragments of the original database along with the corresponding access rights can be specified. For instance, it is possible to select only data of the previous day or the prescribed medication of a patient. Thus, the sensitive data within the EAV storage solution is protected.

4   Evaluation

This section presents some evaluation results for querying the data in the entity-attribute-value storage system. We implemented our EAV storage system using Oracle Database 11.2.0 and Java SE 6. Currently, we are inserting all values into the *String_Value* table. For evaluation, we chose one query, which basically returns all entity-attribute-value tuples in the database. To reconstruct the exact position of an entity in the document, the ancestors and their position among the siblings need to be considered. Therefore, we use a Common Table Expression within a Materialized View to recursively compose the whole ancestor path for an entity. The entity path is composed of the ancestors' names along with their sibling position. An example of one resulting tuple in the form of {entity path, attribute, value} is given below:

{/ClinicalDocument[00]/recordTarget[09]/patientRole[00], classCode, PAT}

We ran a time measurement test five times with two different scenarios: with 10 documents inserted (twice) and with 100 documents inserted (three times). Each test consisted of 10 consecutive runs. The results are shown in table 1. We split up the measured time into three sections: *Before Querying* which mainly includes getting the connection to the database, *Querying* which represents the actual query execution time and *After Querying* which mainly consists of traversing the result set. Due to the caching mechanisms of the database system, the last nine runs of each test were significantly faster in the first two sections than the first run[1]. Hence, the first run as well as the average of all the ten runs in one test are shown.

With only 10 documents in the database, most of the measured time was used before querying with at most 500 ms. The measured time for querying was below 20 ms. Compared to that, the main impact in the scenario with 100 documents can be seen in the performance after querying. The measured time was around 3 seconds which is due to the amount of tuples (39,584) that have to be traversed within the result set. However, we don't expect queries to deliver this amount of tuples in the real application scenario. The performance before querying was similar to the one in the scenario with 10 documents. The measured time for the actual query was between 18 and 29 ms in the first run and therefore at most only 50% higher than in the scenario with 10 documents.

Table 1. Evaluation Results: Time Measured in Milliseconds

Test No	Before Querying		Querying		After Querying	
	First Run	Average	First Run	Average	First Run	Average
1 (10 docs)	478	464.5	15	17	5	4.1
2 (10 docs)	488	126.1	18	4.1	3	1.1
3 (100 docs)	452	122.8	29	4.3	2745	2624
4 (100 docs)	479	124.6	27	4	2693	2588.8
5 (100 docs)	566	152.8	18	3.1	2987	2855.4

---

[1] Surprisingly, the caching mechanism didn't seem to influence any run of the first test. However, the following analysis focuses on the worst case scenario for caching: the first runs. Therefore, this special occurance was not investigated further.

We conclude that the measured time for executing the actual query is by far the lowest compared to the measurements before and after the query. It slightly increases with the number of documents. The time needed before querying is independent from the query and the number of documents in the database.

These results only reflect one query for getting all tuples. An evaluation with attribute-centric queries is part of our future work. Although we know that these queries are less efficient on EAV structured data, the results of the first evaluation are promising.

5   Conclusions and Future Work

In home healthcare, it is very important that information is provided instantly. The heterogeneity of the available systems, i.e., a lack of interoperability, inhibits a fast and flexible exchange of information.

The common standards for exchanging documents in health care are rather generic. Therefore, an adequate storage structure should be also generic in order to handle the heterogeneous data. In this paper, a fundamental database schema based on the Entity-Attribute-Value paradigm is introduced. A mapping of medical documents to this schema can be simply obtained extracting particular information from the document. On the other hand, the generation of standardized documents from the data in the database is considered to be more difficult.

Many other applications use the EAV model for a uniform representation of heterogeneous data. Some of them only offer a search functionality for the data stored in the EAV model. Our approach adds another functionality. By offering an export service, we transform the data in the EAV database into different target formats. Thus, the EAV model is used as the global schema of a heterogeneous federated database architecture. The EAV database is mainly appropriate for this task because of its characteristics: it is able to handle heterogeneous data, and at the same time it allows for future extensions.

The flexibility and dynamic of the entity-attribute-value approach is an important advantage. However, the disadvantage is a possible performance problem at the query processing. A first evaluation showed positive results regarding the performance time for a general query. Further investigations need to be conducted with attribute-centric queries, though. Nevertheless, we can expect the amount of patient data to be relatively small within our scenario. Hence, we expect the impact of attribute-centric queries on performance to be relatively low. Another method to possibly increase the performance is to introduce special index structures, which should also be investigated.

The future work also comprises the definition of views including the development of a role concept for accessing the stored information. Furthermore, the described export transformation process needs to be implemented. The complexity of this process arises from the definition of transformation rules to map the data from the entity-attribute-value structure into the required information in the target format.

References

1. Bortis, G.: Experiences with Mirth: An Open Source Health Care Integration Engine. In: ICSE 2008, pp. 649–652. ACM, New York (2008)
2. Chen, R.S., Nadkarni, P., Marenco, L., Levin, F., Erdos, J., Miller, P.L.: Exploring Performance Issues for a Clinical Database Organized Using an Entity-Attribute-Value Representation. JAMIA 7(5), 475–487 (2000)
3. Corwin, J., Silberschatz, A., Miller, P.L., Marenco, L.: Dynamic Tables: An Architecture for Managing Evolving, Heterogeneous Biomedical Data in Relational Database Management Systems. JAMIA 14(1), 86–93 (2007)
4. Dinu, V., Nadkarni, P., Brandt, C.: Pivoting approaches for bulk extraction of Entity-Attribute-Value data. Computer Methods and Programs in Biomedicine 82(1), 38–43 (2006)
5. Flemming, D., Hübner, U., Heitmann, K.U., Oemig, F., Thun, S.: Implementierungsleitfaden "ePflegebericht" auf Basis der HL7 Clinical Document Architecture Release 2 (2010)
6. Friedman, C., Hripcsak, G., Johnson, S.B., Cimino, J.J., Clayton, P.D.: A Generalized Relational Schema for an Integrated Clinical Patient Database. In: Proc. Annu. Symp. Comput. Appl. Med. Care, pp. 335–339 (1990)
7. Heitmann, K.U., Kassner, A., Gehlen, E., Görke, H.-J., Heidenreich, G.: VHitG Arztbrief - Auf Basis der HL7 Clinical Document Architecture Release 2 (2006)
8. Hellesø, R., Lorensen, M., Sorensen, L.: Challenging the information gap - the patients transfer from hospital to home health care. I. J. of Medical Informatics 73(7-8), 569–580 (2004)
9. Hägglund, M., Scandurra, I., Moström, D., Koch, S.: Integration Architecture of a Mobile Virtual Health Record for Shared Home Care. In: Proceedings of MIE 2005, vol. 116, pp. 340–345 (2005)
10. ISO. EN ISO 21090 Health Informatics - Harmonized data types for information interchange. Technical report, ISO/CEN (2011)
11. Lenz, R., Beyer, M., Kuhn, K.A.: Semantic integration in healthcare networks. I. J. of Medical Informatics 76(2-3), 201–207 (2007)
12. Lenz, R., Beyer, M., Meiler, C., Jablonski, S., Kuhn, K.A.: Informationsintegration in Gesundheitsversorgungsnetzen. Informatik-Spektrum 28, 105–119 (2005), doi:10.1007/s00287-005-0467-4
13. Nadkarni, P.M., Marenco, L., Chen, R., Skoufos, E., Shepherd, G., Miller, P.: Organization of Heterogeneous Scientific Data Using the EAV/CR Representation. JAMIA 6(6), 478–493 (1999)
14. Neumann, C.P., Lenz, R.: α− Flow: A Document-Based Approach to Interinstitutional Process Support in Healthcare. In: Rinderle-Ma, S., Sadiq, S., Leymann, F. (eds.) BPM 2009. LNBIP, vol. 43, pp. 569–580. Springer, Heidelberg (2010)
15. Sunyaev, A., Schweiger, A., Leimeister, J.M., Krcmar, H.: Software-Agenten zur Integration von Informationssystemen im Gesundheitswesen. In: Multikonferenz Wirtschaftsinformatik (2008)
16. Umblia, T., Hein, A., Bruder, I., Karopka, T.: MARIKA: A Mobile Assistance System for Supporting Home Care. In: MobiHealthInf (2009)

Median Polish with Power Transformations as an Alternative for the Analysis of Contingency Tables with Patient Data

Frank Klawonn[1,2], Katja Crull[3], Akiko Kukita[4], and Frank Pessler[5]

[1] Department of Computer Science
Ostfalia University of Applied Sciences
Salzdahlumer Str. 46/48, D-38302 Wolfenbuettel, Germany
[2] Bioinformatics and Statistics
Helmholtz Centre for Infection Research
Inhoffenstr. 7, D-38124 Braunschweig, Germany
[3] Department of Molecular Immunology
Helmholtz Centre for Infection Research
Inhoffenstr. 7, D-38124 Braunschweig, Germany
[4] Department of Microbiology
Saga Medical School
Saga, Japan
[5] Department of Infection Genetics
Helmholtz Centre for Infection Research
Inhoffenstr. 7, D-38124 Braunschweig, Germany

Abstract. Contingency tables are a very common basis for the investigation of effects of different treatments or influences on a disease or the health state of patients. Many journals put a strong emphasis on p-values to support the validity of results. Therefore, even small contingency tables are analysed by techniques like t-test or ANOVA. Both these concepts are based on normality assumptions for the underlying data. For larger data sets, this assumption is not so critical, since the underlying statistics are based on sums of (independent) random variables which can be assumed to follow approximately a normal distribution, at least for a larger number of summands. But for smaller data sets, the normality assumption can often not be justified.

Robust methods like the Wilcoxon-Mann-Whitney-U test or the Kruskal-Wallis test do not lead to statistically significant p-values for small samples. Median polish is a robust alternative to analyse contingency tables providing much more insight than just a p-value.

In this paper we discuss different ways to apply median polish to contingency tables in the context of medical data and how to interpret the results based on different examples. We also introduce a technique based on power transformations to find a suitable transformation of the data before applying median polish.

1   Introduction

Contingency tables often arise from collecting patient data and from lab experiments. The rows and columns of a contingency table correspond to two different categorical

J. He et al. (Eds.): HIS 2012, LNCS 7231, pp. 25–35, 2012.

attributes. One of these categorical attributes could account for different drugs with which patients are treated and the other attribute could stand for different forms of the same disease. Each cell of the table contains a numerical entry which reflects a measurement under the combination of the categorical attributes corresponding to the cell. In the example above, these entries could be the number of patients that have been cured from the disease by the drug corresponding to the cell. Or it could be the time or average time it took patients to recover from the disease while being treated with the drug.

Table 1. A contingency table

Group	Replicate		
G1	6.39	8.10	6.08
G2	8.95	7.48	6.57
G3	5.61	8.58	5.72
G4	813.70	686.50	691.20
G5	4411.50	3778.90	4565.30
G6	32848.40	28866.00	46984.40

Table 1 shows an example of a contingency table. The rows correspond to six different groups. The columns in this case reflect replicates. The columns correspond to 3 replicates of a gene expression experiment where cultured cells were transfected with increasing amounts of an effector plasmid (a plasmid expressing a protein that increases the expression of a gene contained on a second plasmid, referred to as a reporter plasmid) in the presence or absence of the reporter plasmid. Rows 1-3 constitute the negative control experiment, in which increasing amounts of the effector plasmid were transfected, but no reporter plasmid. The experiments in rows 4-6 are identical to those in 1-3, except that increasing amounts of the reporter plasmid were co-transfected. The data correspond to the intensity of the signal derived from the protein which is expressed by the reporter plasmid.

A typical question to be answered based on data from a contingency table is whether the rows or the columns show a significant difference. In the case of the treatment of patients with different drugs for different diseases, one could ask whether one of the drugs is more efficient than the other ones or whether one disease is more severe than the other ones. For the example of the contingency table 1, one would be interested in significant differences among the groups, i.e. the rows. But it might also be of interest whether there might be significant differences in the replicates, i.e. the columns. If the latter question had a positive answer, this could be a hint to a batch effect, which turn out to be a serious problem in many experiments [1].

Hypothesis tests are a very common way to carry out such analysis. One could perform a pairwise comparison of the rows or the columns by the t-test. However, the underlying assumption for the t-test is that the data in the corresponding rows or columns originate from normal distributions. For very large contingency tables, this assumption is not very critical, since the underlying statistics will be approximately normal, even if the data do not follow a normal distribution. Non-parametric tests like the Wilcoxon-Mann-Whitney-U test are a possible alternative. However, for very small contingency tables they cannot provide significant p-values. In any case, a correction for multiple testing – like Bonferroni (see for instance [2]), Bonferroni-Holm [3] or false discovery rate (FDR) correction [4] – needs to be carried in the case of pairwise comparisons.

Instead of pairwise comparisons with correction for multiple testing, analysis of variance (ANOVA) is often applied instead of the t-test. Concerning the underlying model assumptions, ANOVA is even more restrictive than the t-test, since it does even assume that the underlying normal distributions have identical variance. ANOVA is also – like the t-test – very sensitive to outliers. The Kruskal-Wallis test is the corresponding counterpart of the Wilcoxon-Mann-Whitney-U test, carrying out a simultaneous comparison of the medians. But it suffers from the same problems as the Wilcoxon-Mann-Whitney-U test and is not able to provide significant p-values for small samples.

A general question is whether a p-value is required at all. A p-value can only be as good as the underlying statistical model and a lot of information is lost when the interestingness of a whole contingency table is just reflected by a single p-value. In the worst case, a t-test or ANOVA can yield a significant p-value just because of a single outlier.

Median polish [5] – a technique from robust statistics and exploratory data analysis – is another way to analyse contingency tables based on a simple additive model. We briefly review the idea of median polish in Section 2. Although the simplicity of median polish as an additive model is appealing, it is sometimes too simple to analyse contingency table. Very often, especially in the context of gene, protein or metabolite expression profile experiments, the measurements are not taken directly, but are transformed before further analysis. In the case of expression profile, it is common to apply a logarithmic transformation. The logarithmic transformation is a member of a more general family, the so-called power transformations which are explained in Section 3. In this paper, we introduce a method to find a suitable power transformation that yields the best results for median polish for a given contingency table. This idea is introduced in Section 4 and examples are discussed in Section 5, before we conclude the paper.

2   Median Polish

The underlying additive model of median polish is that each entry x_{ij} in the contingency table can be written in the form

$$x_{ij} = g + r_i + c_j + \varepsilon_{ij}.$$

- g represents the overall or grand effect in the table. This can be interpreted as general value around which the data in the table are distributed.
- r_i is the row effect reflecting the influence of the corresponding row i on the values.
- c_j is the column effect reflecting the influence of the corresponding column j on the values.
- ε_{ij} is the residual or error in cell (i, j) that remains when the overall, the corresponding row and column effect are taken into account.

The overall, row and column effects and the residuals are computed by the following algorithm.

1. For each row compute the median, store it as the row median and subtract it from the values in the corresponding row.
2. The median of the row medians is then added to the overall effect and subtracted from the row medians.
3. For each column compute the median, store it as the column median and subtract it from the values in the corresponding column.
4. The median of the column medians is then added to the overall effect and subtracted from the column medians.
5. Repeat steps 1-4 until no changes (or very small changes) occur in the row and column medians.

Table 2 shows the result of median polish applied to Table 1.

Table 2. Median polish for the data in Table 1

	Overall: 350.075			
	R1	R2	R3	row effect
G1	0.000	4.795	−0.310	−343.685
G2	0.000	1.615	−2.380	−341.125
G3	−0.110	5.945	0.000	−344.355
G4	122.500	−1.615	0.000	341.125
G5	0.000	−629.515	153.800	4061.425
G6	0.000	−3979.315	14136.000	32498.325
column effect	0.000	−3.085	0.000	

The result of median polish can help to better understand the contingency table. In the ideal case, the residuals are zero or at least close to zero. Close to zero means in comparison to the row or column effects. If most of the residuals are close to zero, but only a few have a large absolute value, this is an indicator for outliers that might be of interest. Most of the residuals in Table 1 are small, except the ones in the lower right part of the table.

The row effect shows how much influence each row, i.e. in the example, each group has. One can see that group G1, G2 and G3 have roughly the same effect. Group G5 and G6 have extremely high influence and show very significant effects.

The column effects are interpreted in the same way. Since the columns represent replicates, they shall have no effect at all in the ideal case. Otherwise, some batch effect might be the cause. The column effects in Table 1 are – as expected – all zero or at least close to zero.

3   Power Transformations

Transformation of data is a very common step of data preprocessing (see for instance [6]). There can be various reasons for applying transformations before other analysis steps, like normalisation, making different attribute ranges comparable, achieving certain distribution properties of the data (symmetric, normal etc.) or gaining advantage for later steps of the analysis.

Power transformations (see for instance [5]) are a special class of parametric transformations defined by

$$t_\lambda(x) \;=\; \begin{cases} \frac{x^\lambda - 1}{\lambda} & \text{if } \lambda \neq 0, \\ \ln(x) & \text{if } \lambda = 0. \end{cases}$$

It is assumed that the data values x to be transformed are positive. If this is not the case, a corresponding constant ensuring this property should be added to the data.

We restrict our considerations on power transformations that preserve the ordering of the values and therefore exclude negative values for λ.

In the following section, we use power transformation to improve the result of median polish.

4   Finding a Suitable Power Transformations for Median Polish

An ideal result for median polish would be when all residuals are zero or at least small. The residuals get smaller automatically when the values in the contingency table are smaller. This would mean that we tend to put a high preference on the logarithmic transformation ($\lambda = 0$), at least when the values in the contingency table are greater than 1. Small for residuals does not refer to the absolute values of the residuals being small. It means that the residuals should be small compared to the row or column effects. Therefore, we should compare the absolute values of the residuals to the absolute values of the row or column effects. One way to do this would be to compare the mean values of the absolute values of the residuals to the mean value of the absolute values of the row or column effects. This would, however, be not consistent in the line of robust statistics. Single outliers could dominate this comparison. This would also lead to the reverse effect as considering the residuals alone. Power transformations with large values for λ would be preferred, since they make larger values even larger. And since the row or column effects tend to be larger than the residuals in general, one would simply need to choose a large value for λ to emphasize this effect.

Neither single outliers of the residuals nor of the row or column effects should have an influence on the choice of the transformation. What we are interested in is being able to distinguish between significant row or column effects and residuals. Therefore, the spread of the row or column effects should be large whereas at least most of the absolute values of the residuals should be small.

To measure the spread of the row or column effects, we use the interquartile range which is a robust measure of spread and not sensitive to outliers like the variance. The interquartile range is the difference between the 75%- and the 25%-quantile, i.e. the range that contains 50% percent of the data in the middle.

We use the 80% quantile of the absolute values of all residuals to judge whether most of the residuals are small. It should be noted that we do not expect all residuals to be small. We might have single outliers that are of high interest.

Finally, we compute the quotient of the interquartile range of the row or column effects and divide it by the 80% quantile of the absolute values of all residuals. We call this quotient the IQRoQ value (**InterQuartile Range** over the 80% **Quantile** of the absolute residuals). The higher the IQRoQ value, the better is the result of median polish. For each value of λ, we apply the corresponding power transformation to the contingency table and calculate the IQRoQ value. In this way, we obtain an IQRoQ plot, plotting the IQRoQ value depending on λ.

Of course, the choice of the interquartile range – we could also use the range that contains 60% percent of the data in the middle – and the 80%-quantile for the residuals are rules of thumb that yield good results in our applications. If more is known about the data, for instance that outliers should be extremely rare, one could also choose a higher quantile for the residuals.

Before we come to examples with real data in the next section, we illustrate our method based on artificially generated contingency tables. The first table is a 10×10, generated by the following additive model. The overall effect is 0, the row effects are $10, 20, 30, \ldots, 100$, the column effects are $1, 2, 3, \ldots, 10$. We then added to each entry noise from a uniform distribution over the interval $[-0.5, 0.5]$ to each entry.

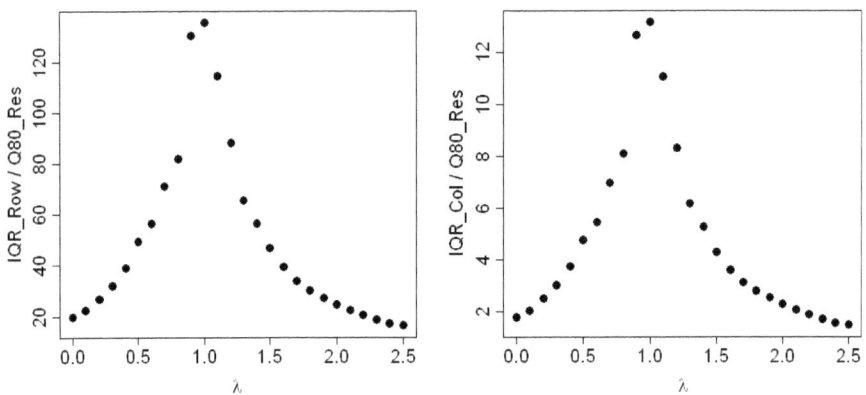

Fig. 1. IQRoQ plot for the row (left) and column effects (right) for the artificial example data set

Figure 1 shows the IQRoQ plots for the row and column effects for this artificial data set. In both cases, we have a clear maximum at $\lambda = 1$. So the IQRoQ plots propose to apply the power transformation with $\lambda = 1$ which is the identity transformation and leaves the contingency table as it is. The character of the IQRoQ plots for the row and column effects is similar, but the values differ by a factor 10. This is in complete accordance with the way the artificial data set had been generated. The row effects were chosen 10 times as large as the column effects.

As a second artificial example we consider the same contingency table, but apply the exponential function to each of its entries. The IQRoQ plots shown in Figure 2 have their maximum at $\lambda = 0$ and therefore suggest to use the logarithmic transformation before applying median polish. So this power transformation reverses the exponential function and we retrieve the original data which were generated by the additive model.

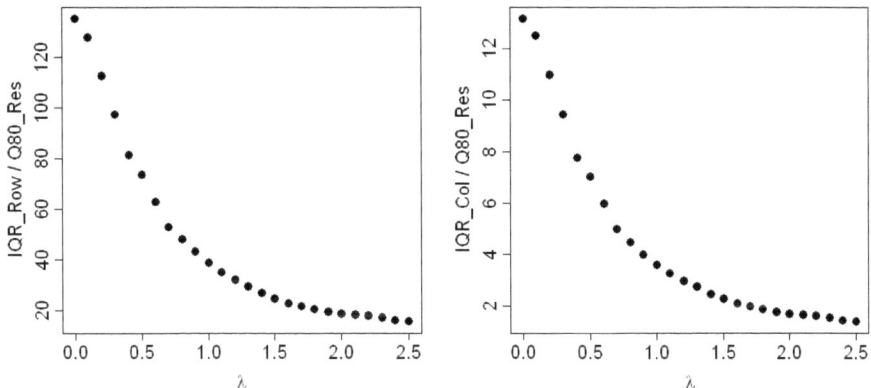

Fig. 2. IQRoQ plot for the row (left) and column effects (right) for the exponential artificial example data set

The last artificial example is a negative example in the sense that there is no additive model underlying the data generating process. The entries in the corresponding 10×10 contingency table were produced by a normal distribution with expected value 5 and variance 1. The IQRoQ plots are shown in Figure 3. The IQRoQ plot for the row effect has no clear maximum at all and shows a tendency to increase with increasing λ. The IQRoQ plot for the column effect has a maximum at 0 and then seems to oscillate with definitely more than one local maximum. There is no clear winner among the power transformations. And this due to the fact that there is no underlying additive model for the data and no power transformation will make the data fit to an additive model.

5   Examples

We now apply the IQRoQ plots to real data sets. As a first example, we consider the data set in Table 1. The IQRoQ plots are shown in Figure 4. The IQRoQ plot for the row effects has its global maximum at $\lambda - 0$ and a local maximum at $\lambda = 0.5$. The IQRoQ plot for the column effects has its global maximum at $\lambda = 0.5$. However, we know that in this data set the columns correspond to replicates and it does not make sense to maximise the effects of the replicates over the residuals. The IQRoQ values for the column effects are also much smaller than the IQRoQ values for the row effects. Therefore, we chose the power transformation suggested by the IQRoQ plot for the row effects, i.e. the logarithmic transformation induced by $\lambda = 0$. The second choice would be the power transformation with $\lambda = 0.5$ which would lead to similar effects as the logarithmic transformation, although not so strong.

Table 3 shows the result of median polish after the logarithmic transformation has been applied to the data in Table 1. We compare this table with Table 2 which originated from median polish applied to the original data. In Table 3 based on the optimal transformation derived from the IQRoQ plots, the absolute values of all residuals are

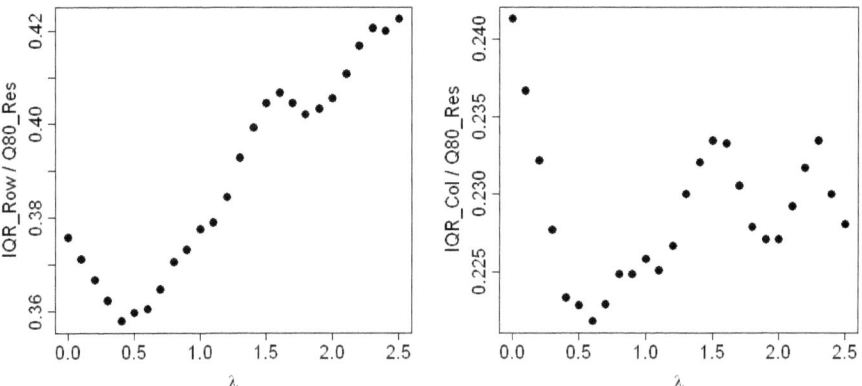

Fig. 3. IQRoQ plot for the row (left) and column effects (right) for a random data set where all entries in the contingency table were generated by a normal distribution with expected value 5 and variance 1

Table 3. Median polish for the data in Table 1 after power transformation with $\lambda = 0$

	R1	R2	R3	row effect
Overall: 4.2770				
G1	0.0000	0.2422	−0.0497	−2.4223
G2	0.1760	0.0017	−0.1331	−2.2614
G3	−0.0194	0.4106	0.0000	−2.5331
G4	0.1632	−0.0017	0.0000	2.2614
G5	0.0000	−0.1497	0.0343	4.1149
G6	0.0000	−0.1241	0.3579	6.1226
column effect	0.0000	−0.0051	0.0000	

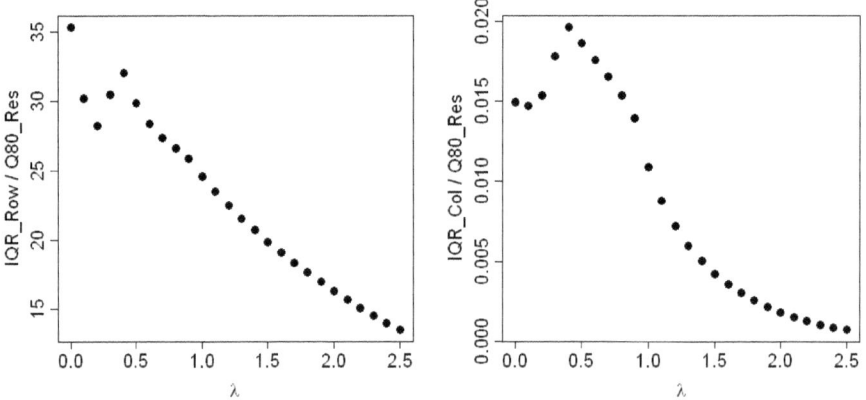

Fig. 4. IQRoQ plot for the row (left) and column effects (right) for the data set in Table 1

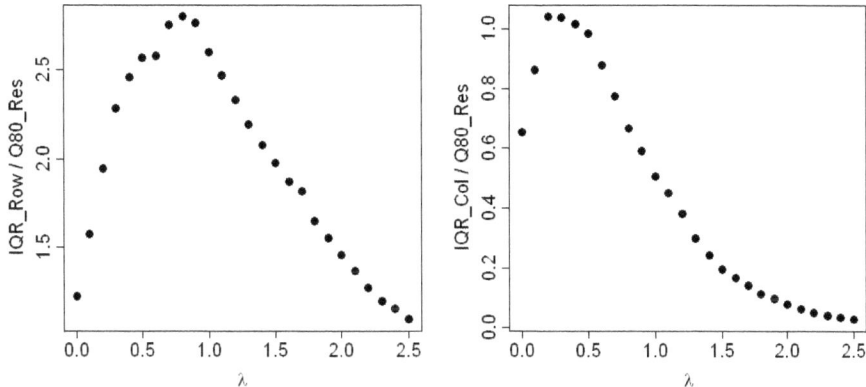

Fig. 5. IQRoQ plot for the row (left) and column effects (right) for a larger contingency table for spleen

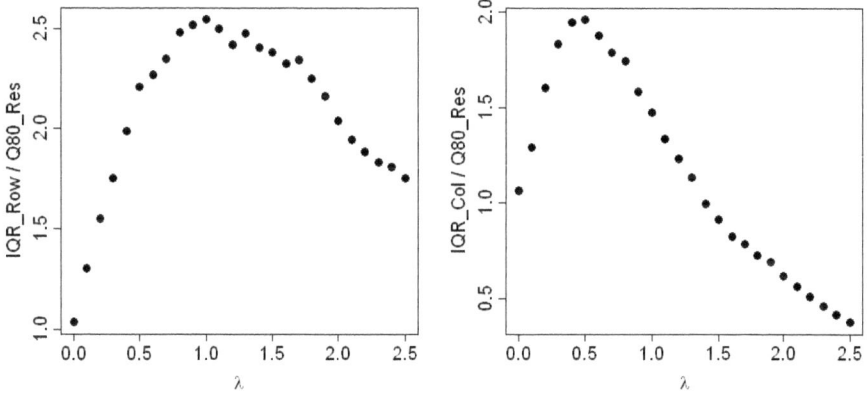

Fig. 6. IQRoQ plot for the row (left) and column effects (right) for a larger contingency table for tumour

smaller than any of the (absolute) row effects. There is no indication of extreme outliers anymore, whereas the median polish in Table 2 applied to the original data suggests that there are some extreme outliers. The entries for G6 for replicate R2 and R3 and even the entry for G5 for replicate R2 show a larger absolute value of the majority of the row effects in Table 2. From Table 2, it is also not very clear whether group G4 is similar to groups G1, G2, G3 or groups G5, G6, whereas after the transformation in Table 1 the original groupings G1, G2, G3 (no reporter plasmid) versus of G4, G5, G6 (with increasing amount of reporter plasmid) can be easily identified based on the row effects.

We finally consider two larger contingency tables with 14 rows and 97 columns that are far too large to be included in this paper. The tables consist of a data set displaying the metabolic profile of a bacterial strain after isolation from different tissues of a mouse. The columns reflect the various substrates whereas the rows consist of repetitions for the isolates from tumor and spleen tissue. The aim of the analysis is to identify those substrates that can be utilized by active enzymes and to find differences in the metabolic profile after growth in different organs.

The corresponding IQRoQ plots are shown in Figures 5 and 6. The IQRoQ plots indicate that we choose a value of around $\lambda = 0.5$, although the IQRoQ plots do not agree on exactly the same value.

6   Conclusions

We have introduced a method to select a power transformation to improve the results of median polish. The method has been illustrated by artificial examples as well as by example based on real data. Choosing the right power transformation can give a much clearer picture of the median polish result than the median polish directly applied to the raw data.

IQRoQ plots or values can also be used when only a limited number of power transformations would be meaningful for a given data set. For instance, one could either want to analyse the raw data ($\lambda = 1$) or the data after logarithmic transformation ($\lambda = 0$). Then it is not necessary to generate full IQRoQ plots. It is then sufficient to just calculate the two IQRoQ values and choose the power transformation that yields the higher values.

Future studies will include a sensitivity analysis of the choice of the quantile for the residuals on which the IQRoQ value is based. The proposed 80% quantile seems to be a good choice, but further studies are required to confirm this conjecture.

7   Program Code

The IQRoQ plots in this paper were generated by an implementation of the described method in R, a free software environment for statistical computing and graphics [7] (see http://www.r-project.org/). The simple R implementation for generating IQRoQ plots can be downloaded at

http://public.ostfalia.de/~klawonn/medpol_powertrans.R

Acknowledgements. This study was co-financed by the European Union (European Regional Development Fund) under the *Regional Competitiveness and Employment* objective and within the framework of the Bi^{2}SON Project *Einsatz von Informations- und Kommunikationstechnologien zur Optimierung der biomedizinischen Forschung in Südost-Niedersachsen.*

References

1. Leek, J., Scharpf, R., Corrado Bravo, H., Simcha, D., Langmead, B., Johnson, W., Geman, D., Baggerly, K., Irizarry, R.: Tackling the widespread and critical impact of batch effects in high-throughput data. Nature Reviews|Genetics 11, 733–739 (2010)

2. Shaffer, J.P.: Multiple hypothesis testing. Ann. Rev. Psych. 46, 561–584 (1995)
3. Holm, S.: A simple sequentially rejective multiple test procedure. Scandinavian Journal of Statistics 6, 65–70 (1979)
4. Benjamini, Y., Hochberg, Y.: Controlling the False Discovery Rate: A Practical and Powerful Approach to Multiple Testing. Journal of the Royal Statistical Society. Series B (Methodological) 57, 289–300 (1995)
5. Hoaglin, D., Mosteller, F., Tukey, J.: Understanding Robust and Exploratory Data Analysis. Wiley, New York (2000)
6. Berthold, M., Borgelt, C., Höppner, F., Klawonn, F.: Guide to Intelligent Data Analysis: How to Intelligently Make Sense of Real Data. Springer, London (2010)
7. R Development Core Team: R: A Language and Environment for Statistical Computing. R Foundation for Statistical Computing, Vienna, Austria (2009)

An Integrated Approach for Healthcare Planning over Multi-dimensional Data Using Long-Term Prediction

Rui Henriques and Cláudia Antunes

D2PM, IST–UTL, Portugal
{rmch,claudia.antunes}@ist.utl.pt

Abstract. The mining of temporal aspects over multi-dimensional data is increasingly critical for healthcare planning tasks. A healthcare planning task is, in essence, a classification problem over health-related attributes across temporal horizons. The increasingly integration of healthcare data through multi-dimensional structures triggers new opportunities for an adequate long-term planning of resources within and among clinical, pharmaceutical, laboratorial, insurance and e-health providers. However, the flexible nature and random occurrence of health records claim for the ability to deal with both structural attribute-multiplicity and arbitrarily-high temporal sparsity. For this purpose, two solutions using different structural mappings are proposed: an adapted multi-label classifier over denormalized tabular data and an adapted multiple time-point classifier over multivariate sparse time sequences. This work motivates the problem of long-term prediction in healthcare, and places key requirements and principles for its accurate and efficient solution.

1 Introduction

New planning opportunities are increasingly triggered by the growing amount, quality and integration of healthcare data through multi-dimensional structures. Research in classification over healthcare domains has been focused on early diagnosis, series description and treatment selection [5]. The mining of temporal dynamics have been mainly applied over physiological signals, with few additional methods over sequential genomic and proteomic structures.

Dealing with temporal aspects in broader contexts represents an unprecedented opportunity for healthcare planning. An example is the task of planning hospital resources by predicting if a patient will need a specific treatment within upcoming periods. For this task, a multi-dimensional structure centered in health records is commonly adopted [29]. Although there are mappings to temporal and tabular structures for the ready-application of classifiers, as illustrated in Fig.1, the resultant temporal event-sparsity and attribute-multiplicity trigger the need for a new understanding and formulation. Additionally, challenges of long-term prediction in the healthcare include the ability to deal with different time scales [1][5], advanced temporal rules [23] and knowledge-based constraints for an accurate and efficient long-term learning with minimum domain-specific noise [3].

J. He et al. (Eds.): HIS 2012, LNCS 7231, pp. 36–48, 2012.
© Springer-Verlag Berlin Heidelberg 2012

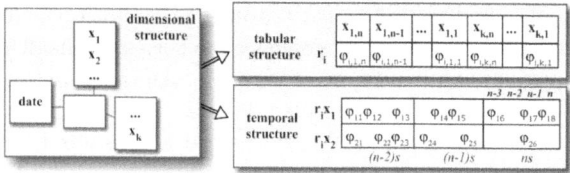

Fig. 1. Structural mappings to apply long-term predictors

The document is structured as follows. Section 2 introduces the current challenges of healthcare planning tasks. In sections 3 and 4, the problem of long-term prediction over multi-dimensional structures is motivated and formulated. Section 5 places key requirements for its accurate and efficient solution. Finally, an overview of the relevant work in long-term prediction is synthesized.

2   Healthcare Planning Challenges

Healthcare planning tasks include improvement of care pathways, detection of inefficiencies, resources allocation, health trends retrieval, and study of drug reactions and treatment effects. These applications have the potential to improve health, increase patient satisfaction and reduce costs. Similarly to predictive medicine, planning models can personalize guidelines to the characteristics of a single patient [5]. However, the assessment of his current state does not suffice. Evolving behavior across temporal horizons needs to be present.

2.1   Integrated Healthcare Data

In the last decade, new patient-centric data sources emerged. Countries as United Kingdom and Netherlands, already track patients' movements across health providers, payors and suppliers. The changing landscape has been shaped by: *i)* consumer-pushed demand through direct-access to risk and diagnosis information outside of the hospital setting, *ii)* new requirements for drug and treatment development, *iii)* the use of expert-systems to support medical decisions for quality compliance, and *iv)* remote home monitoring.

The stakeholders of healthcare planning are: *i)* data generators as hospitals, clinics, payors, pharmacies, e-prescription companies, laboratories and diagnostic-services providers; *ii)* data collectors as e-record vendors; and *iii)* data analyzers as pharmacos, application vendors and the research community.

Datasets are increasingly less fragmented, with appearing both cross-country and cross-player offerings, as provided by Cegedim and IMS. Datasets are derived from claims (Ingenix, D2Hawkeye, CMS), e-health records (McKesson, GE, PracticeFusion), imported health records (GoogleHealth, HealthVault), content aggregators (Walters Kluer, Reed Elsevier, Thomson), patient communities (Alere, Pharos, SilverLink, WebMD, HealthBoards), consumer reports (Anthem, vimo, hospitalcompare), online worksite healthcare (iTrax, webConsult), and physician portals (Medstory, Sermo, Doctors.net.uk).

This work uses health records as the mean to organize the wide variety of episodes into a single and compact fact [29]. In order to deal with record data flexibility, which may include laboratory results, prescriptions, treatments, diagnostics, free-text and complex structures as time series, an health record defines what the fact represents and the type of its fields. Amounts are mined as ordinal symbols, free-text is ignored, and complex data is converted into categorical sets of symbols. In Fig.2, an illustrative health record is presented.

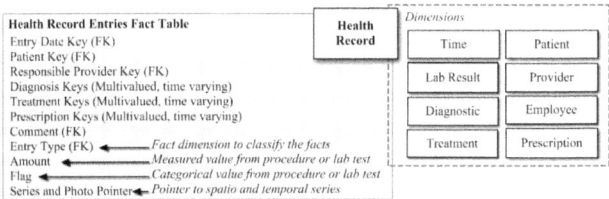

Fig. 2. Health record-centered multi-dimensional structure

2.2   Emerging Challenges

The increasing integration and volume of healthcare data trigger new challenges in terms of learning efficiency, attribute multiplicity and occurrence sparsity. These challenges are synthesized in Table 1.

Table 1. Critical requirements of healthcare planning

Predictor requirement	Healthcare data properties
Methods to deal with missing values and event sparsity	Health records are irregularly collected due to an uneven schedule of visits or measurements made;
Strategies to deal with multivariate structures	Health records can flexibly define a high-multiplicity of attributes (e.g. wearables can produce measures for more than 20 attributes);
Efficient structural operations for record alignment and temporal partitioning	Health records' sampling grid varies both within and across patients;
Calendric-pattern discovery and aggregation techniques to deal with the different sampling rate of health records	Physiological measurements may be continuously generated, while administrative records as time-stamped prescriptions or hospitalizations exist at a coarser scale;
Convolutional memory techniques and pattern-based learning ability to detect evolving health trends	Evolutionary patterns, as the slow progress of a disorder or a reaction to a prescription or treatment, are spread across many potentially non-relevant health records;
Background knowledge guidance to avoid efficiency and domain-noise problems	The number of health records can be significantly high and its flexible nature hampers the learning;

3   A Need for a Novel Long-Term Prediction Formulation

Given a training dataset of series composed by $n+h$ observations of the form (x,y), where $x=\{\varphi_1,...,\varphi_n\}$ and $y=\{\varphi_{n+1},...,\varphi_{n+h}\}$, the task of traditional *long-term prediction* is to learn a predictive model to label the h next observations, where $h > 1$ is the *prediction horizon*.

This definition enters the scope of long-term prediction over series of elements. Since this work targets multi-dimensional structures characterized by multivariate and non-equally distant observations, there is the need to understand existing approaches and to incrementally extend this definition.

3.1 Limitations of Long-Term Prediction over Tabular Structures

A simple way to deal with long-term prediction over multi-dimensional structures is to denormalize them into plain tabular structures. The long-term prediction task over tabular data can be target by an adapted multi-label classifier, as illustrated in Fig.3a. The goal of multi-label classification is to learn a model from an input dataset to predict a set of attributes whose class label is unknown.

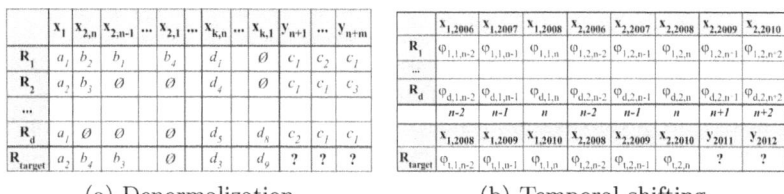

(a) Denormalization   (b) Temporal shifting

Fig. 3. Long-term prediction over tabular data

This option has several challenges. *First*, its viability strongly depends on the ability to represent the predicting horizon as attributes, and on the temporal compliance with the dataset instances. *Second*, by capturing each health record as a set of attributes, the size of the table may grow dramatically, which can significantly reduce the efficiency of the learning process and the accuracy of the classification model. *Third*, multi-label classifiers are neither prone to deal with ordinal attributes nor to capture the temporal dependencies among them. To solve these challenges, adaptations to multi-label classifiers are required to consider temporal dynamics and to constrain the learning over large datasets.

3.2 Limitations of Long-Term Prediction over Temporal Structures

Let us assume that a mapping between a multi-dimensional and a temporal structure is possible, as illustrated in Fig.4. Let time sequences be the target temporal structure, as they do not put constraints on the arriving distribution of events. With this formulation, three challenges arise. The *first* challenge is of adapting predictors to deal with arbitrary-high sparse time sequences. When mapping multi-dimensional data to time sequences, the rate of health records' occurrence per patient and across patients may vary significantly. Structural sparsity results from the alignment of records across time points. Additionally, a mapping between a multi-dimensional dataset into non-temporal sequences would only consider events' precedences (Fig.4). Thus, existing learners are not ready for time-sensitive prediction over time sequences.

The *second* challenge is of dealing with multivariate time sequences. Each arriving health record can be seen as a vector of optional attributes. When considering the task of predicting long-term hospitalizations, the attribute under prediction can be the first vector position, while the remainder vector positions correspond to optional prescriptions, symptoms, exams and diagnostics. These adjunct attributes may influence the attribute under prediction (determining

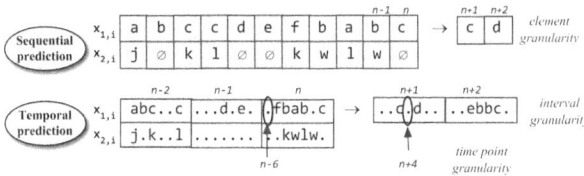

Fig. 4. Sequential and temporal prediction over time sequences

if either a patient is hospitalized or not) and, therefore, are not conditionally independent from the attribute under prediction. At a finer granular level, vector positions can be physiological measures. Research on multivariate responses has been focusing on projecting multivariate attribute in the form of a matrix of responses, but assuming independence among them [31][12].

The *third* challenge is of performing long-term prediction in evolving contexts. Its relevance in planning problems is discussed in [20]. Different problems can be identified depending on the adopted predictor. Predictors can either scan local or large partitions depending, respectively, whether the time sequence is considered non-stationary or stationary. When considering local partitions nothing but cyclic behavior can be mined. When large partitions are considered and a lazy learner is adopted, over-fitting and pattern-negligence can arise. Alternatively, by adopting a non-lazy approach, the learner has to collapse all the predictive ability within a model. In this case, smoothing is an undesirable but possible result in order to avoid model complexity and over-fit propensity. The understanding of evolutionary patterns, beyond cyclic and calendric patterns, may be required to complement the learning [40]. An evolutionary pattern, as an evolving disease, can either be a subsequence whose occurrence is not cyclic but dependent on a time function or a cyclic subsequence whose arrangement progressively changes. The mining of evolutionary aspects can increase prediction accuracy, particularly for time-points near the horizon of prediction.

4   Problem Formulation

Conventional predictors define a multiple-input single-output mapping. In *iterated* methods [6], a h-step-ahead prediction problem is tackled by iterating h times the one-step-ahead predictor. Taking estimated values as inputs, instead of actual observations, has negative impact in error propagation [44][39]. *Direct* methods learn h models, each returning a direct forecast. Although not prone to the accumulation of prediction errors [44], they require higher complexity to model the stochastic dependencies between non-similar series. Additionally, the fact that the n models are learned independently:

$$P(y|x) = P(\{\varphi_{n+1}, ..., \varphi_{n+h}\} \mid x) = \Pi_{i=1}^{h} P(\varphi_{n+i} \mid x),$$

prevents this approach from considering underlying dependencies among the predicted variables that may result in a biased learning [9][39].

Multiple-Input Multiple-Output (MIMO) methods learn one multiple-output predictive model. This favors efficiency and preserves the stochastic dependencies for a reduced bias, even though it reduces the flexibility of single-output approaches that may result in a new bias [9][6]. To avoid this, *Multiple-Input Several Multiple-Outputs* (MISMO) uses intermediate configurations to decompose the original task into $k = h/s$ prediction tasks, where h is the prediction horizon and s is the size of horizon's partitions. This approach trades off the property of preserving the stochastic dependency among future values with a greater flexibility of the predictor [50].

Definition 1. *Single-output* approaches either predict $\hat{\varphi}_i$: *i)* directly: $f_{i \in \{1,...,h\}}$ $(\varphi_n, .., \varphi_{n-d})$, where h is the prediction horizon, d is a subset of total observations (embedding dimension), and f is the stochastic predictor; or *ii)* iteratively as $f_{i \in \{1,..,h\}} = \{f_{i=1}(\varphi_n, ..., \varphi_{n-d}), f_{i \in \{2,...,d-1\}}(\hat{\varphi}_{n+i-1}, ..., \hat{\varphi}_{n+1}, \varphi_n, ..., \varphi_{n-d+i}),$ $f_{i \in \{d,...,h\}}(\hat{\varphi}_{n+i-1}, ..., \hat{\varphi}_{n+i-d})\}$. *Multiple-output* approaches predict the $h=ks$ time-points within k steps $\{\varphi_{n+ps}, ..., \varphi_{n+(p-1)s+1}\} = f_p(\varphi_n, \varphi_{n-1}, ..., \varphi_{n-d+1}),$ with $p \in \{1, ..., k\}$, where s, the predictor's variance, constrains the perseveration of stochastic properties of the series, null if $s=1$ and maximal if $s=n$.

4.1   Tabular Formulation

Definition 2. Consider a training dataset consisting of a set of m instances of the form $(x_1, ..., x_n, y_1, ...y_h)$, such that $(y_1, .., y_h) \in Y$ is either a numeric or a categorical vector $(Y=\mathbb{R}^h | \Sigma^h)$; and each x_i takes on values from a domain $X_i = \cup_k \{(\Sigma_i | \mathbb{R}, k)\}$, where $k \in \mathbb{N}$ defines the event occurrence's order. The task of **long-term prediction over tabular data** is to construct either a single-output or multiple-output mapping model $M : \{X_1, ..., X_n\} \rightarrow Y$ for the multi-period classification of new tuples.

Using a multi-dimensional dataset, of we want to predict the number of hospitalizations for a patient j over a period i, y_i^j, we need to perform three steps. *First*, to use the patient dimension to select the health records per instance, x^j, based on patient primary key. *Second*, to use the time dimension for its ordering. *Finally*, to denormalize the health record measures in n attributes. For instance, using blood pressure measures, an example of patient j attributes is $x^j = \{x_{highbp}^j, x_{lowbp}^j\}$, with $x_{highbp}^j = \{(10, t_1), (9, t_2), (11, t_3), (\emptyset, t_4), .., (\emptyset, t_{max})\}$, and $x_{lowbp}^j = \{(7, t_1), (5, t_2), (7, t_3), (\emptyset, t_4), .., (\emptyset, t_{max})\}$.

4.2   Time Sequence Formulation

Considering a *sampling interval* $\tau \in \mathbb{R}$ and the *alphabet* Σ:

Definition 3. A **time series** with regard to a series of equally-distant time points, $\mathbb{I} = \{\theta_1, ..., \theta_m\}$ with $\{\theta_i = \tau_0 + i\tau; i \in \mathbb{R}\}$ of length $m \in \mathbb{N}$, is $z = \{(\theta_i, \varphi_i) \mid \varphi_i = [\varphi_{i,1}, ..., \varphi_{i,d}]^T \in (\Sigma | \mathbb{R})^d, i=1, ..., n\}$. A **time sequence** is a multi-set of events, $z = \{(\varphi_i, \theta_j) \mid \varphi_i = [\varphi_{i,1}, ..., \varphi_{i,d}]^T \in (\Sigma | \mathbb{R})^d; i=1, ..., n; j \in \mathbb{N}^+\}$. z is univariate if $d=1$ and **multivariate** if $d>1$.

Considering the illustrative sparse time sequence $x = \{([10\ 7], \theta_1), ([\emptyset\ \emptyset], \theta_2), ([\emptyset\ \emptyset], \theta_3), ([9\ 5], \theta_4), ([13\ 7], \theta_5)$ composed of $d=2$ multivariate observations across $n=5$ time points. Long-term prediction consists of using a dataset of similar time sequences to predict a class of interest across $h=p \times s$ periods.

Definition 4. Given a training dataset consisting of m instances of the form $(x, y_1, .., y_h)$, where $x=\{(\varphi_1, \theta_1), .., (\varphi_n, \theta_n)\} \in X$ is a time sequence of n-length and $y \in Y$ is a univariate time series a set of h-length, the task of **longterm prediction over multivariate and sparse temporal structures** is to construct either a single-output model or multiple-output model $M : X \to Y$, where $h>1$ and $\varphi_i = [\varphi_{i,1}, .., \varphi_{i,d}]^T$ with $d>1$.

The process of mapping a multi-dimensional dataset into a multivariate time sequence differs from the previous on the third step. The time dimension is now used to distribute the events' occurrence according to a timeline, instead of a simple ordering. The definition of aggregating functions as the average, sum or count, can be used for events' composition in coarser-granular time scales.

4.3 Problem Generalization

Depending on the availability of training tuples compliant with the temporal horizon of prediction and on the allowance of temporal shifts, we may benefit to transit from a pure supervised solution into an hybrid one. Fig.3b illustrates a case where a 2-year shift is required. If significant noise results from this action, additional semi-supervised and unsupervised principles are required [40][1][51].

4.4 Evaluation

The evaluation of long-term predictors requires different metrics than those used in traditional classification. The *accuracy* of a predictive model is the probability that the predictor correctly labels multiple time points, $P(\hat{y}=y)$.

When the class for prediction is ordinal, the accuracy of the long-term predictor should be based on a similarity function. The average normalized root mean squared error (NRMSE) and the symmetric mean absolute percentage of error (SMAPE) have been employed in the literature. If the class for prediction is nominal, the similarity function should be replaced by the intersection operator.

$$NRMSE(y, \hat{y}) = \frac{1}{h} \frac{\Sigma_{i=1}^h \sqrt{(y_i - \hat{y}_i)^2}}{y_{max} - y_{min}} \quad SMAPE(y, \hat{y}) = \frac{1}{h} \Sigma_{i=1}^h \frac{|y_i - \hat{y}_i|}{(y_i + \hat{y}_i)/2} \ [6]$$

$$Accuracy_{ord} = \frac{1}{m} \Sigma_{j=1}^m 1 - (NRMSE(y^j, \hat{y}^j) \mid SMAPE(y^j, \hat{y}^j))$$

$$Accuracy_{nom} = \frac{1}{m} \Sigma_{j=1}^m (\frac{1}{h} \Sigma_{i=1}^h \mid y_i^j \cap \hat{y}_i^j \mid)$$

Predictor's *efficiency* should be measured in terms of memory consumed and time elapsed for both the training (model learning) and prediction stages.

Finally, complementary metrics to understand the predictor's *error accumulation* [15] and *smoothness* [15], when noise fluctuations are present, should be adopted for a deeper understanding of the predictor's behavior.

5   Solution Space

Key variables, illustrated in Fig.5, must be considered to solve the introduced requirements of long-term prediction in healthcare planning.

For instance, the *target data* variable is dependent on the health records' representation, degree of sparsity, noise sensitivity, completeness, length, degree of content-stationarity, presence of static features, multivariate order, patterns presence, attributes' alphabet amplitude, and sensitivity to temporal shifts.

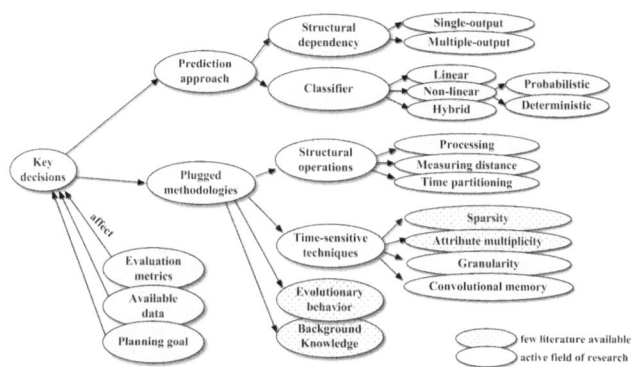

Fig. 5. Key research areas for long-term prediction

5.1   Adopted Learning Approach

Several implementations for both single-output and multiple-output approaches exist. All of them, implicitly or explicitly, work around the multivariate conditional distribution $P(Y|X)$. Learners can either follow linear or non-linear predictive models. *Linear models* can either follow a simple, logistic or Poisson regression, as auto-regressions and feed-forward moving average mappings [33].

Non-linear long-term predictors can either define probabilistic or deterministic models. Most are adaptations of traditional classifiers using temporal sliding windows. Probabilistic predictors include (hidden) conditional random fields [28]; hidden and variable-memory Markov models (HMM) [34][4]; and stochastic grammars [14]. Deterministic predictors include support vector machines (SVM) [13]; recurrent, time-delay and associate neural networks [24][8][30]; multiple adaptive regression splines [35]; regression and model trees [11][42]; multiple lazy learning alternatives [9]; and genetic solvers [16].

5.2   Plugged Methodologies

Despite the relevance of the learning approach choice, the significant performance improvements is triggered by the temporal criteria that predictors may adopt [40]. Since the learning of long-term predictors are NP-hard [38], the understanding of efficient structural operations, time-based strategies, temporal rules and knowledge-based constraints is key.

Structural Operations. Suitable data representations [19], similarity-measures [19] and time-partitioning strategies are required for a quick and flexible learning. Criteria for temporal partitioning through clustering, user-defined granularities, fuzzy characterization, split-based sequential-trees, episodes, domain-driven ontologies and symbolic interleaving can be consulted in [41][38][1].

Time-Sensitive Techniques. Strategies to enhance the performance of long-term predictors for healthcare planning tasks are synthesized in Table 2.

Table 2. Long-term prediction principles and hypotheses

Requirement	Research contributions
data sparsity	Time windows can be adopted to create ordering or temporal partitions [41]. This can be used to constraint the exponential growth of denormalized tables and to selected the most recent health records' occurrences in order to avoid missing values. In time sequences, they can be used for flexible learning approaches, but additional techniques are required to deal with missing values, as proposed in [37][26];
temporal granularity	Different levels of granularity defined using time windows and feature-based descriptions hold the promise of minimizing problems of sparsity and efficiency, even though the data loss can degrade predictors' accuracy. To manage this trade-off, the study of improvements using hierarchical zooming operations [22] and calendars [2] is key;
data attributes multiplicity	Dependencies among attributes have been captured either through the use of additional attributes or by defining weights on how each attribute (e.g. prescription) influences a different attribute (e.g. symptom) across the time horizon [40]. In time sequences, learning strategies can be adopted to deal with sparse multivariate vectors that may constrain the vector under prediction [31]. One option is to project each vector or attribute to the target horizon [12], and to derive from them the vector under prediction;
memory sampling	Covariance functions, following either a parametric or non-parametric approach, are key for the selective forgetting of unimportant events and retaining of decisive events [48]. In both tabular and temporal structures, these functions can assign weights to each attribute or time point to be used by long-term predictors. Binary or exponentially decaying weighted average of an input function can be used to set a trade-off between *depth* (how far back memory goes) and *resolution* (the degree to which information about individual time-points is preserved).

Evolutionary Behavior. Mining of evolutionary behavior, discussed in section 3, is required to avoid smoothing and overfitting problems. An understandable case is prediction rules, which specify a causal and temporal correlation between two time points or patterns. In [20], emerging or evolutionary patterns are defined as patterns whose support increases significantly over time. Although pattern-based classifiers seem a suitable choice, other approaches should not be excluded. Examples may include the late combination of temporal rules within a predictive model or, alternatively, their initial retrieval to assist its learning [41].

Background Knowledge. Finally, background knowledge is increasingly claimed as a requirement for long-term prediction as it guides the definition of time windows [41]; provides methods to bridge different time scales, to treat monitoring holes and to remove domain-specific noise [5]; defines criteria to prune the explosion of multiple-equivalent patterns [3]; and fosters the ability to adapt and incrementally improve results by refining the way domain-knowledge is represented [3]. A hierarchy of flexible sequential constraints, and of relaxations ranging from conservative to distance-based approximations is introduced in [1]. Further research on domain-driven time modeling is required [2].

6 Related Research

Time series long-term prediction and *sequence learning* are the research streams with major relevant contributions for the introduced problem.

Long-Term Prediction. A comparative study on the performance of iterated and direct single-output approaches in terms of error accumulation, smoothness, and learning difficulty is presented in [45]. In literature, *hybrid* solutions that combine both approaches exist [45]. Experimental results in [39] show that the robustness and error reduction obtained using direct and hybrid forecasts do not justify the price paid in terms of increased sampling variance. Values for the MISMO variance parameter can be derived from query-point functions. Experimental studies [50] show that the s best-value strongly varies according dataset, with s=1 (Direct method) and s=n (MIMO method) being good performers in less than 20% of the cases. For large horizons h, improvements in multiple-output approaches have been achieved by adopting operators as the partial autocorrelation [50]. A comparison of five multi-step-ahead prediction methods, two single-output and three multiple-output predictors is done in [6].

Potential linear, probabilistic and deterministic classifiers were discussed. In [15] an hybrid HMM-regression is evaluated using different regression orders and time-windows sizes. Evaluation of three multiple-output neural predictors, simple feed-forward, modular feed-forward and Elman, is done in [7]. In [10], Bayesian learning is applied to recurrent neural networks to deal with noisy and non-stationary time series. In [9][27], multiple-output approaches, as least-squares SVM, are extended with query-based criteria grounded on local learning.

Sequence Learning. Sequence learning methods are adopted when the mining goal is either sequence prediction, sequence recognition or sequential decision making [46]. Sequence recognition can be formulated as a prediction problem.

Learning techniques as expectation maximization, gradient descendant, policy iteration, hierarchical structuring or grammar training can be transversally applied to different implementations [28]. Markov models are the most adopted classification method [21]. Additionally, unsupervised and reinforcement learning techniques from machine learning have been applied to sequence prediction, even though are still not scalable for large data volumes.

First, *unsupervised learning* rely on motifs, calendric rules, episodes, containers and partially-ordered tones [1][40][38] to assist prediction. In [36], patterns are translated into boolean features to guide SVM and logistic regressions.

Second, *reinforcement learning* [49] have been applied in inductive-logic predictors (that learn symbolic knowledge from sequences in the form of expressive rules) [32] and in evolutionary computing predictors (that use heuristic-search over probabilistic models of pattern likelihood) [47]. In [18], sequence-generating rules constrain which symbol can appear. In [17], series are used to train trees, from which rules are retrieved and combined with logical operators.

Finally, a large spectrum of implementations are hybrid. An example is the use of symbolic rules and evolutionary computation applied to neural networks [47]. The introduced reinforcement learning techniques are usually preferred when one is not interested in a specific temporal horizon, but rather in predicting the occurrence of a certain symbol or pattern.

Healthcare Planning. A good survey covering temporal classification advances in healthcare can be found in [5]. In [43], simple planning problems were address relying on administrative health records including drug prescriptions, hospitalizations, outpatient visits, and daily hospital activities. State-based characterization using Markov models were, for instance, applied to predict the risk of stroke in sickle cell anemia patients [5]. Temporal abstractions have been used for multiple time-point classification of physiological signals. In [25], a collaborative approach is designed to mine biomedical multivariate time series to understand vector evolution. The mining of evolving health aspects for planning tasks have, however, received few attention. In [5], its combination with large-scale genomics and proteomics is pointed as a decisive step to characterize disease progression.

7   Conclusion

This work addresses healthcare planning problems using long-term prediction over multi-dimensional structures centered in health records. It introduced two formulations based on structural mappings into tabular structures and multivariate sparse temporal structures. The combination of unsupervised and reinforcement learning techniques should be present when the training and testing tuples are not temporally compliant and sensitive to temporal shifts. Evaluation metrics for the target problem are proposed.

A set of requirements were introduced to deal with attribute multiplicity and temporal-sparsity of health records. Contributions were identified. Literature is either focused on long-term prediction over single-attributes or on causal learning, not answering the introduced challenges. Empirical contributions in the form of principles that satisfy one or more of these requirements are the expected next steps to promote an efficient learning of accurate long-term predictors with minimum domain-specific noise.

Acknowledgment. This work is partially supported by *Fundação para a Ciência e Tecnologia* under the research project D2PM, PTDC/EIA-EIA/110074/2009, and the PhD grant SFRH/BD/75924/2011.

References

1. Antunes, C.: Pattern Mining over Nominal Event Sequences using Constraint Relaxations. Ph.D. thesis, Instituto Superior Tecnico (2005)
2. Antunes, C.: Temporal pattern mining using a time ontology. In: EPIA, pp. 23–34. Associação Portuguesa para a Inteligência Artificial (2007)
3. Antunes, C.: An ontology-based framework for mining patterns in the presence of background knowledge. In: ICAI, pp. 163–168. PTP, Beijing (2008)
4. Begleiter, R., El-Yaniv, R., Yona, G.: On prediction using variable order markov models. J. Artif. Int. Res. 22, 385–421 (2004)
5. Bellazzi, R., Ferrazzi, F., Sacchi, L.: Predictive data mining in clinical medicine: a focus on selected methods and applications. Wiley Interdisc. Rew.: Data Mining and Knowledge Discovery 1(5), 416–430 (2011)

6. Ben Taieb, S., Sorjamaa, A., Bontempi, G.: Multiple-output modeling for multi-step-ahead time series forecasting. Neurocomput. 73, 1950–1957 (2010)
7. Bengio, S., Fessant, F., Collobert, D.: Use of modular architectures for time series prediction. Neural Process. Lett. 3, 101–106 (1996)
8. Berthold, M., Hand, D.J. (eds.): Intelligent Data Analysis: An Introduction. Springer-Verlag New York, Inc., Secaucus (1999)
9. Bontempi, G., Ben Taieb, S.: Conditionally dependent strategies for multiple-step-ahead prediction in local learning. Int. J. of Forecasting 27(2004), 689–699 (2011)
10. Brahim-Belhouari, S., Bermak, A.: Gaussian process for nonstationary time series prediction. Computational Statistics and Data Analysis 47(4), 705–712 (2004)
11. Breiman, L., Friedman, J.H., Olshen, R.A., Stone, C.J.: Classification and Regression Trees. Chapman & Hall, New York (1984)
12. Brown, P.J., Vannucci, M., Fearn, T.: Multivariate bayesian variable selection and prediction. Journal of the Royal Statistical Society 60(3), 627–641 (1998)
13. Burges, C.J.C.: A tutorial on support vector machines for pattern recognition. Data Min. Knowl. Discov. 2, 121–167 (1998)
14. Carrasco, R.C., Oncina, J.: Learning Stochastic Regular Grammars by Means of a State Merging Method. In: Carrasco, R.C., Oncina, J. (eds.) ICGI 1994. LNCS, vol. 862, pp. 139–152. Springer, Heidelberg (1994)
15. Cheng, H., Tan, P.-N., Gao, J., Scripps, J.: Multistep-Ahead Time Series Prediction. In: Ng, W.-K., Kitsuregawa, M., Li, J., Chang, K. (eds.) PAKDD 2006. LNCS (LNAI), vol. 3918, pp. 765–774. Springer, Heidelberg (2006)
16. Cortez, P., Rocha, M., Neves, J.: A Meta-Genetic Algorithm for Time Series Forecasting. In: Proc. of AIFTSA 2001, EPIA 2001, Porto, Portugal, pp. 21–31 (2001)
17. Cotofrei, P., Neuchâtel, U.: Rule extraction from time series databases using classification trees. In: Proc. of the 20th IASTED, pp. 327–332. ACTA Press (2002)
18. Dietterich, T.G., Michalski, R.S.: Discovering patterns in sequences of events. Artif. Intell. 25, 187–232 (1985)
19. Ding, H., Trajcevski, G., Scheuermann, P., Wang, X., Keogh, E.J.: Querying and mining of time series data: experimental comparison of representations and distance measures. Proceedings of the VLDB Endowment 1(2), 1542–1552 (2008)
20. Dong, G., Li, J.: Efficient mining of emerging patterns: discovering trends and differences. In: 5th ACM SIGKDD, KDD, pp. 43–52. ACM, NY (1999)
21. Eddy, S.R.: Profile hidden markov models. Bioinformatics/Computer Applications in the Biosciences 14, 755–763 (1998)
22. Fang, Y., Koreisha, S.G.: Updating arma predictions for temporal aggregates. Journal of Forecasting 23(4), 275–296 (2004)
23. Freksa, C.: Temporal reasoning based on semi-intervals. A. Int. 54, 199–227 (1992)
24. Guimarães, G.: The Induction of Temporal Grammatical Rules from Multivariate Time Series. In: Oliveira, A.L. (ed.) ICGI 2000. LNCS (LNAI), vol. 1891, pp. 127–140. Springer, Heidelberg (2000)
25. Guyet, T., Garbay, C., Dojat, M.: Knowledge construction from time series data using a collaborative exploration system. J. of Biomedical Inf. 40, 672–687 (2007)
26. Hsu, C.N., Chung, H.H., Huang, H.S.: Mining skewed and sparse transaction data for personalized shopping recommendation. Mach. Learn. 57, 35–59 (2004)
27. Ji, Y., Hao, J., Reyhani, N., Lendasse, A.: Direct and Recursive Prediction of Time Series Using Mutual Information Selection. In: Cabestany, J., Prieto, A.G., Sandoval, F. (eds.) IWANN 2005. LNCS, vol. 3512, pp. 1010–1017. Springer, Heidelberg (2005)
28. Kersting, K., De Raedt, L., Gutmann, B., Karwath, A., Landwehr, N.: Relational Sequence Learning. In: De Raedt, L., Frasconi, P., Kersting, K., Muggleton, S.H. (eds.) Probabilistic ILP 2007. LNCS (LNAI), vol. 4911, pp. 28–55. Springer, Heidelberg (2008)

29. Kimball, R., Ross, M.: The Data Warehouse Toolkit: The Complete Guide to Dimensional Modeling, 2nd edn. John Wiley & Sons, Inc., NY (2002)
30. Kleinfeld, D., Sompolinsky, H.: Associative neural network model for the generation of temporal patterns: Theory and application to central pattern generators. Biophysical Journal 54(6), 1039–1051 (1988)
31. Koch, I., Naito, K.: Prediction of multivariate responses with a selected number of principal components. Comput. Stat. Data Anal. 54, 1791–1807 (2010)
32. Lavrac, N., Dzeroski, S.: Inductive Logic Programming: Techniques and Applications. Ellis Horwood, New York (1994)
33. Laxman, S., Sastry, P.S.: A survey of temporal data mining. Sadhana-academy Proceedings in Engineering Sciences 31, 173–198 (2006)
34. Laxman, S., Sastry, P.S., Unnikrishnan, K.P.: Discovering frequent episodes and learning hidden markov models: A formal connection. IEEE Trans. on Knowl. and Data Eng. 17, 1505–1517 (2005)
35. Lee, T.S., Chiu, C.C., Chou, Y.C., Lu, C.J.: Mining the customer credit using classification and regression tree and multivariate adaptive regression splines. Computational Statistics & Data Analysis 50(4), 1113–1130 (2006)
36. Lesh, N., Zaki, M.J., Ogihara, M.: Mining features for sequence classification. In: Proc. of the 5th ACM SIGKDD, pp. 342–346. ACM, NY (1999)
37. Liu, J., Yuan, L., Ye, J.: An efficient algorithm for a class of fused lasso problems. In: Proc. of the 16th ACM SIGKDD, KDD, pp. 323–332. ACM, NY (2010)
38. Mannila, H., Toivonen, H., Inkeri Verkamo, A.: Discovery of frequent episodes in event sequences. Data Min. Knowl. Discov. 1, 259–289 (1997)
39. Marcellino, M., Stock, J.H., Watson, M.W.: A comparison of direct and iterated multistep ar methods for forecasting macroeconomic time series. Journal of Econometrics 135(1-2), 499–526 (2006)
40. Mörchen, F.: Time series knowledge mining. W. in Dissertationen, G&W (2006)
41. Mörchen, F.: Tutorial cidm-t temporal pattern mining in symbolic time point and time interval data. In: CIDM. IEEE (2009)
42. Quinlan, J.R.: Learning with continuous Classes. In: 5th Australian Joint Conf. on Artificial Intelligence, pp. 343–348 (1992)
43. Silberschatz, A., Tuzhilin, A.: What makes patterns interesting in knowledge discovery systems. IEEE Trans. on Knowl. and Data Eng. 8, 970–974 (1996)
44. Sorjamaa, A., Hao, J., Reyhani, N., Ji, Y., Lendasse, A.: Methodology for long-term prediction of time series. Neurocomput. 70, 2861–2869 (2007)
45. Sorjamaa, A., Lendasse, A.: Time series prediction using dirrec strategy. In: ESANN, pp. 143–148 (2006)
46. Sun, R., Giles, C.L.: Sequence learning: From recognition and prediction to sequential decision making. IEEE Intelligent Systems 16, 67–70 (2001)
47. Sun, R., Peterson, T.: Autonomous learning of sequential tasks: experiments and analyses. IEEE Transactions on Neural Networks 9(6), 1217–1234 (1998)
48. Sutton, R.S.: Learning to predict by the methods of temporal differences. Machine Learning 3, 9–44 (1988)
49. Sutton, R., Barto, A.: Reinforcement learning: an introduction. Adaptive computation and machine learning. MIT Press (1998)
50. Taieb, S.B., Bontempi, G., Sorjamaa, A., Lendasse, A.: Long-term prediction of time series by combining direct and mimo strategies. In: Proc. of the 2009 IJCNN, pp. 1559–1566. IEEE Press, Piscataway (2009)
51. Wang, W., Yang, J., Muntz, R.: Temporal association rules on evolving numerical attributes. In: Proc. of the 17th ICDE, pp. 283–292. IEEE CS, USA (2001)

A Novel Automated Recognition System Based on Medical Machining CAD Models

Hao Lan Zhang, Weitao Jiang, Huiqin Wu, and Libing Shu

Ningbo Institute of Technology, Zhejiang University
Ningbo, Zhejiang, China, 315100
haolan.zhang@nit.zju.edu.cn,
{jiangwt2007,huiqinwood}@163.com,
shulibing@gmail.com

Abstract. CAD/CAM software products can help boost productivity for machining medical parts. However, the process of evaluating and re-calculating CAD model design is basically carried out manually. The demand for automated CAD process systems has been rising. Automated feature recognition (AFR) systems can improve system efficiency and effectiveness for processing CAD models in manufacturing sectors, particularly for designing medical machining parts. However, existing AFR methods are unable to fulfill industrial requirements for extracting and recognizing domain components from CAD models efficiently. In this paper we suggest a knowledge-based AFR system that can efficiently identify domain components from CAD models. The AFR knowledgebase incorporates rule-based methods for identifying core components from CAD models. The process of defining the rules and fact base structure is one of the most critical issues in the AFR system design. There is no existing technology available for generating inference rules from the STEP model format. The AFR-based system has successfully solved the technical issues in both the inference process and STEP-based extraction process. The skeleton software has been successfully developed based on the modularized system framework. The skeleton software can effectively recognize the common domain specific components.

Keywords: CAD Model Design, Medical Machining Parts Analysis, Knowledge-based systems.

1 Introduction

The range of medical components are very broad, from the parts assembled into a hospital bed to the tiny bone screw used to hold pieces of the body together in surgery [1]. Therefore, a computer-based machining process is essential for improving the medical components design.

This research project addresses the specific problem occurred in the medical CAD model design analysis process, which mainly relies on the human-based FR process.

J. He et al. (Eds.): HIS 2012, LNCS 7231, pp. 49–59, 2012.
© Springer-Verlag Berlin Heidelberg 2012

The human-based FR process is time-consuming, cost-ineffective, and inaccurate. The demand for an effective AFR system is rising in the manufactory sector, particularly in the aerospace sector. Current AFP applications adopt knowledge-based methodologies as the most common solution for FR process.

Knowledge-based AFR systems utilize various artificial intelligent techniques to solve the problems in the recognition processes. Numerous FR applications have been developed through incorporating existing feature recognition methods into knowledge-based systems [2, 3, 4, 5, 6]. However, most of the existing FR applications are unable to integrate with a CAD database that contains design description of the part including geometry details and topological information [5]. This limitation could cause many problems in FR processes such as the lack of accuracy, lack of consistency, time consuming, etc.

This project investigates existing FR methods and proposes a knowledge-based AFR system for medical parts design analysis. The following figures show the CAD models of medical parts [7].

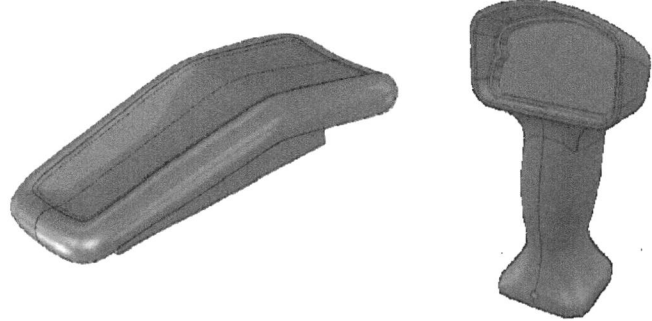

Fig. 1. CAD Model of Medical Machining Parts [7]

2   Related Work

Numerous FR methods have been suggested in the last two decades. However, only few of them have been widely used in academic research and industry applications. The most common methods used in various AFR applications include:

- Rule-based FR,
- Hint based FR,
- Graph-based FR,
- Artificial neural network-based FR.

These feature recognition methods should be distinguished from the specific feature extraction techniques in terms of acquiring geometric data. The following examples show how rules can be applied to the AFR system:

Rule-1: IF $(45° \leq$ (Face_A ∩ Face_X$_i$) $\leq 135°$) &
(Face_A is_surrounded_by {Face_X$_i$}) &
(Face_A is Plane)
THEN (Face_A ∈ PANEL SUPPORT)

Rule-2: IF $(45° \leq$ Face_A ∩ Face_X$_i$ $\leq 135°$) &
(Face_Xi ∈ PANEL SUPPORT) &
(Face_A ∈ Face_X$_i$ _bounded_Faces_Set {Face-i})
THEN (Face_A ∈ STIFFENER SUPPORT)

Rule-3: IF (Edge_A ∈ Face_X$_1$) &
(Edge_A ∈ Face_X$_2$) &
THEN (Face_X$_1$ ∩ FaceX$_2$)

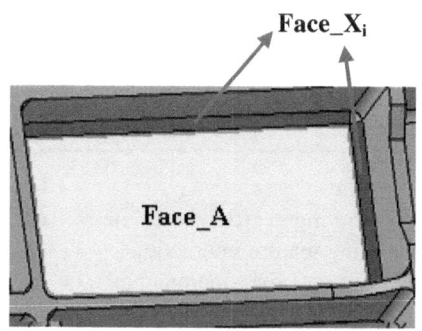

Fig. 2. Example AFR Rules for CAD Model Design

Rule-based FR method is the most common and efficient solution for various FR systems [3, 8]. It has proven to be a robust method, which can handle more recognition objects than other syntactic methods [3]. The general structure of rule-based systems separates rules and facts, which enhances the system flexibility and rationality.

The graph-based method of feature recognition recognizes features by representing geometric and topological information of a design part as a graph, applying graph isomorphism algorithms to match feature patterns to pre-defined sub-graphs [9, 10].

An Artificial Neural Network (ANN) is composed of a number of nodes, or units, connected by links. Each link has a numeric weight associated with it [11, 12].

The selection of an appropriate FR method is crucial to the success of a FR system. Therefore, conducting a comparison of existing FR methods would help us to apply proper FR methods to the AFR system. Table 1 briefly illustrates the comparison of four major FR methods mentioned in the previous sections; and also includes the volumetric decomposition FR method.

Some research work has incorporated these recognition methods into a hybrid method [12], which inspires the knowledge-based design of the AFR system.

Table 1. Comparison of Existing FR Methods

FR Method	Advantages	Disadvantages
Rule-based	• Offering direct, explicit, and rational representation, • High level of independency, • Enhancing flexibility, • Supporting other FR methods.	• Lack of self-training capability, • Lack of efficiency for handling feature interactions.
Hint-based	• Capable for recognizing more complex features, • Improving accuracy (compared to a solely FR method).	• Inexplicit recognition, • Large info process, • Lack of self-training capability.
Graph-based	• Improving efficiency of solving feature interactions, • Effective for incremental feature modeling.	• Causing combinatorial explosion problems, • Unable to solve graph isomorphism problems.
Artificial Neural Network	• Supporting supervised and unsupervised training • Improving FR accuracy • Reducing rule base size and avoiding exhaustive searching • Supporting high-level feature inference (rather than in geometry levels)	• Unable to deal with semantic descriptions • Lack of rationality (poor knowledge representation) • Difficulty of generating appropriate training sets

3   AFR System Design Process

3.1   AFR Work Process and Data Flow Diagram

The first step for the AFR system is to identify the AFR work process flowchart, which is derived from the SPAT-based work process and incorporating the rule-based FR method. The AFR work process flowchart consists of five phases including the knowledge interpretation phase, AFR initialisation phase, AFR extraction phase, AFR recognition phase, and finalisation phase.

The second essential method employed for analyzing and constructing the AFR system framework is AFR Data Flow Diagram (DFD). Based on the AFR work process flowchart, the DFD of the AFR system can be generated for clarifying the system structure and design processes as shown in Figure 3. The DFD entities in the AFR system mainly consist of domain experts and system users. The illustrations of these two types of DFD entities help AFR system developers to understand the desired inputs and outputs. Thus, the AFR system can be designed more efficiently to accommodate the needs of these two types of external entities.

The knowledge interpretation phase involves in managing AFR rules, domain knowledge, and constraints. In this phase, domain experts can define, modify, and update AFR rules that can be further used by the feature extraction and recognition phases.

The AFR initialisation phase is focused on setting the initial parameters for the AFR rule-based system, such as the area value of panels, angles between panels and stiffeners, edge loop numbers, etc. This phase also allows system users to import CAD models to the AFR system.

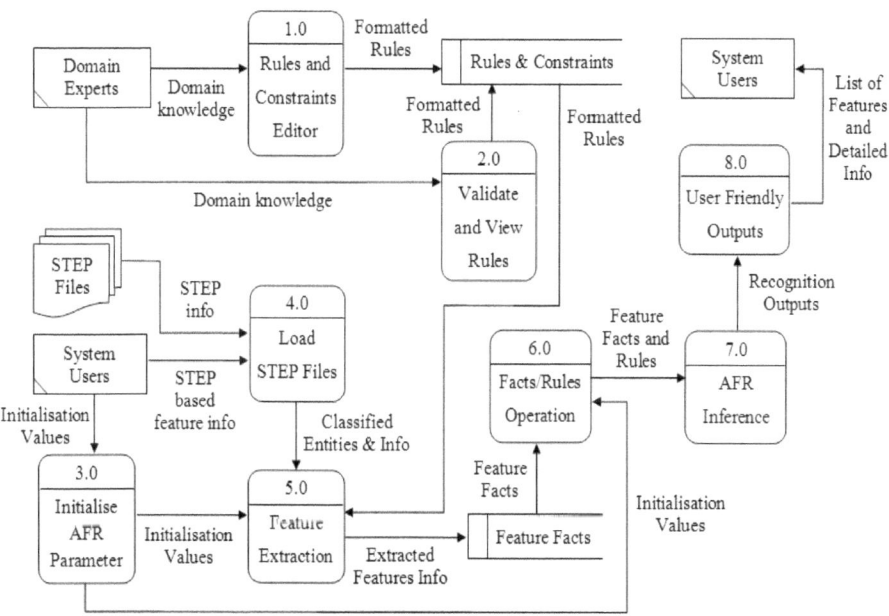

Fig. 3. Data Flow Diagram of the AFR System

The AFR recognition phase employs optimised FR algorithms to replace the human-based recognition process. This phase incorporates the domain knowledge from the knowledge interpretation phase, which converts the domain experts' knowledge to AFR rules and other knowledge-based forms, such as attributed adjacency graphs. The inference process will search and match the classified CAD entities against AFR rules and constraints to identify the domain specific components. The recognition process will associate the relationships between domain components based and CAD entities based on the inference results.

The finalisation phase generates user-friendly outputs, which will provide detailed topological and geometrical information to system users.

The knowledge interpretation phase involves in managing AFR rules, domain knowledge, and constraints. In this phase, domain experts can define, modify, and update AFR rules that can be further used by the feature extraction and recognition phases. The AFR initialisation phase is focused on setting the initial parameters for the AFR rule-based system. This phase also allows system users to import CAD models to the AFR system. Several knowledge based methods have been incorporated into the AFR extraction and recognition phase to replace the human-based recognition process. In this phase, the domain expert knowledge is converted to AFR rules, fact bases, and other knowledge-based forms. The inference process will search and match the classified CAD entities against AFR rules and constraints to identify the domain specific components.

The finalisation phase generates user-friendly outputs, which will provide detailed topological and geometrical information to system users.

3.2   Knowledge-Based System in AFR

A Knowledge-based System (KBS) is a computer system that utilises artificial intelligence methods to solve domain problems. The core components of a KBS are the knowledge base and the inference mechanisms. Expert systems, case-based reasoning systems and neural networks are all particular types of knowledge-based systems.

Basically, a KBS consists of three major phases as shown in Figure 4. The acquisition process obtains knowledge inputs from external environment (generally domain experts), and passes the acquired knowledge to the next phase. The representation phase represents and stores the acquired knowledge in the knowledge base through a logical and explicit way, which can be interpreted by computers. The inference process generates the reasoning results based on the knowledge base, and delivers the results to external environment (generally systems users) as outputs.

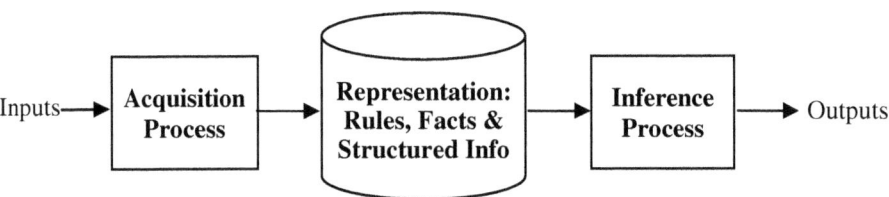

Fig. 4. Three Major Processes of KBS

KBSs have been applied extensively to various industrial sectors particularly the manufacturing sector including medical machining parts [14, 15]. The applications of KBSs in the manufacturing design process could produce benefits for design and manufacturing processes, which include: reducing time-consumption and manpower, improving system accuracy and efficiency, maximising system flexibility and adaptability through knowledge sharing and structured knowledge representation. These factors motivate the application of KBS techniques to the AFR system.

Knowledge representation techniques are mainly concerned with the representation of domain knowledge in structured and explicit ways. Knowledge representation techniques address the knowledge from two major aspects, i.e. the declarative knowledge and procedural knowledge. The declarative knowledge represents the domain entities or facts, and general relationships between these facts, and constraints. This type of knowledge is also interpreted as 'what' knowledge [15]. The procedural knowledge defines the procedures of generating and obtaining facts, relationships, etc., in order to find solution to specific problems. The major knowledge representation techniques are listed as follows.

- Semantic networks: A semantic network or net is a graphic notation for representing knowledge in patterns of interconnected nodes and arcs [16]. It is a network, which represents semantic relations between the concepts. This KR technique has been deployed extensively in various applications, such as WordNet database, Gellish dictionary, etc., as one of the major KR techniques. A semantic network is a declarative graphic representation that can be used either to represent knowledge or to support automated systems for reasoning about knowledge [16].
- Frames and scripts: A frame-based KR can be viewed as a predefined semantic network, which contains a set of slots containing names or values. Frames consists of value slots, for instance, the frame for 'car' might contain a 'manufacturer' slot, 'number of door' slot. Scripts are a type of frame that describes what happens temporally. Scripts use a series of related frames to represent dynamic information as a sequence a stereotypic events.
- Ontology-based representation: Ontology is a data model that represents a set of concepts within a domain, and the relationships between those concepts. It is used to reason about the objects within that domain. Ontology describes formally a domain of discourse. Different from databases, which mainly concerning storing data, ontology specifies a representational vocabulary for a shared domain – definitions of classes, functions, and other objects. Ontology represents the conceptual structure and internal/external relationships of an entity. Ontologies are used in artificial intelligence, the semantic web, software engineering, biomedical informatics, and information architecture as a form of knowledge representation about the world or some part of it.

4   Three-Level of AFR Knowledge-Base

The domain level knowledge defines domain specific components, such as stiffeners, panels, etc., and domain specific rules and constraints. The task knowledge specifies what facts and associated information should be generated, which include the structures of neutral CAD format files, STEP files in particular, and the modelling rules. The process knowledge specifies detailed functions and processes for obtaining information specified in task knowledge level. The following figures show the AFR knowledge base framework based on the three level of knowledge.

Domain knowledge level: The domain specific information of a stiffened-panel model can be described through feature definitions and incorporate AFR rules for domain-specific components. The domain knowledge in the AFR knowledge base generally refers to the engineering domain (particularly in the stiffened panels design area).

Task knowledge level: The task knowledge in the AFR knowledge base is used to establish models for CAD entities. This enables the inference process to identify 'what' knowledge used in the AFR process as shown in Figure 5.

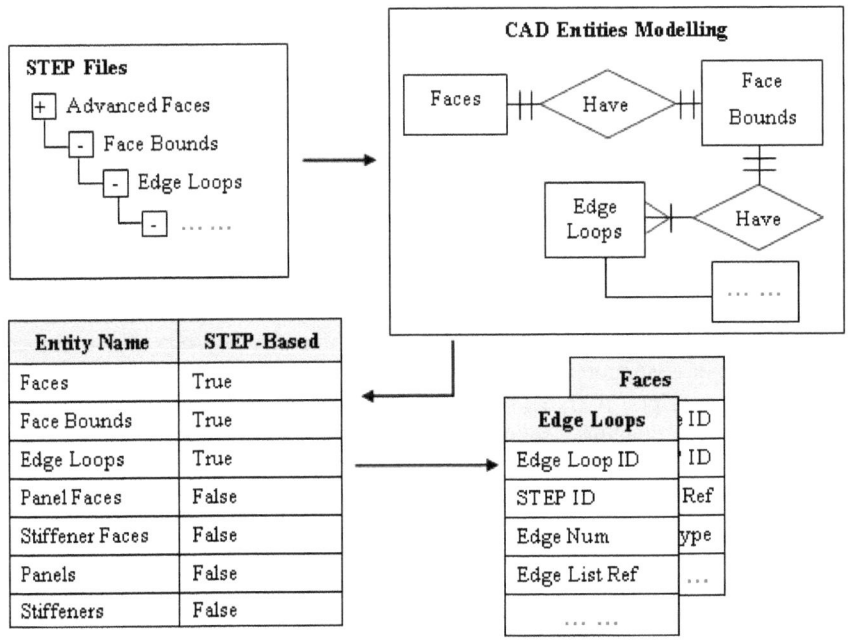

Fig. 5. An Example of AFR Task Knowledge

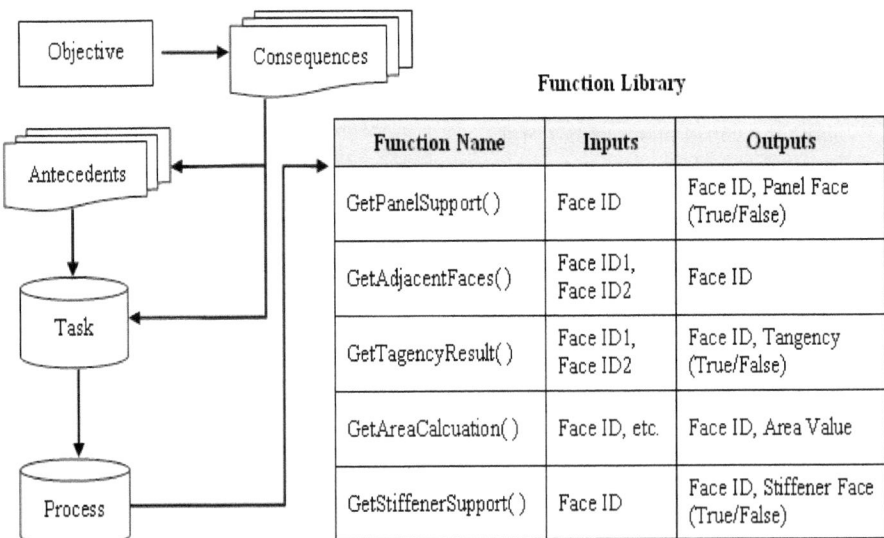

Fig. 6. An Example of AFR Process Knowledge

Process knowledge level: This level provides procedure information about 'how' to obtain the details specified in the task knowledge as shown in Figure 6.

An editor application has been developed with a Graphical User Interface (GUI) accommodating fields for specifying system knowledge. The interface of the KBS editor design is illustrated in Figure 7.

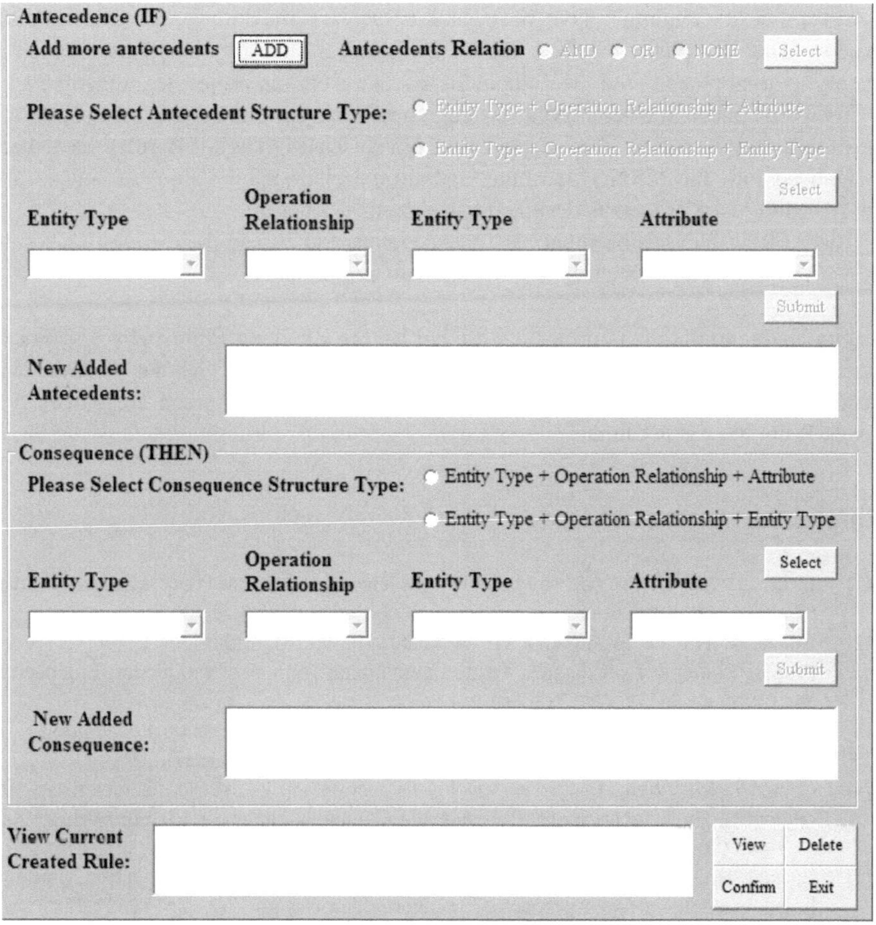

Fig. 7. KBS Editor Application of AFR

5   Conclusion

This research reviews and clarifies the procedures and techniques used in designing the AFR knowledge base for automated recognition of medical CAD models. The AFR knowledge acquisition and representation process explores and analyses various techniques for constructing the AFR systems, and establishes the AFR knowledge base framework. The AFR knowledge base construction process has gone through five phases, which include: FR methods review phase, design process investigation phase, typical cases selection phase, KA phase, and KR phase.

The ontological view of the AFR knowledge base has been represented in three levels of knowledge including the domain knowledge, task knowledge, and process knowledge. Each level of knowledge addresses specific aspects of designing AFR knowledge base.

Several KA techniques have been used to acquire the knowledge from domain experts. The KA phase overlaps the design process investigation phase, which is mainly focused on acquired the domain knowledge from the project team members.

In the KR phase, the acquired knowledge has been represented in a formulised and structured way based on the selected two typical cases. The AFR rules have been formulised into the "Entity-Attribute-Operation Relationship-Value" structure; and the AFR inference process is designed based on this structure.

The AFR system has been successfully developed [17]; and the recognition results show the system can efficiently identify domain components.

Acknowledgements. This project is funded by the Zhejiang Philosophy and Social Science Project Fund (Grant No. 11JCSH03YB), Overseas Scholar Science and Technology Excellent Project Funding 2011 (Ministry of Human Resources and Social Security of P.R China).

References

[1] Fishman, H.: CAD/CAM for Medical Machining. Delcam Press Release, Delcam Copyright (2009)

[2] Bouzakis, H.K.D., Andreadis, G.: A Feature-based Algorithm for Computer Aided Process Planning for Prismatic Parts. International Journal of Production Engineering and Computers 3(3), 17–22 (2000)

[3] Babic, B., Nesic, N., Miljkovic, Z.: A Review of Automated Feature Recognition With Rule-based Pattern Recognition. Computers in Industry 59, 321–337 (2008)

[4] Chen, Y.-M., Wen, C.-C., Ho, C.T.: Extraction of geometric characteristics for manufacturability assessment. Robotics and Computer-Integrated Manufacturing 19(4), 371–385 (2003)

[5] Lockett, H.L., Guenov, M.D.: Graph-based Feature Recognition for Injection Moulding based on a Mid-surface Approach. Computer-Aided Design 37(2), 251–262 (2005)

[6] Yuen, C.F., Wong, S.Y., Venuvinod, P.K.: Development of a Generic Computer-Aided Process Planning Support System. Journal of Materials Processing Technology 139, 394–401 (2003)

[7] Global Inspection Solution. "3D Scanning", Corporate Documentation, Global Spection Solution (2007)

[8] Sadaiah, M., Yadav, D.R., Mohanram, P.V., Radhakrishnan, P.: A Generative CAPP System for Prismatic Components. International Journal of Advanced Manufacturing Technology 20, 709–719 (2002)

[9] Jones, T.: Automated Feature Recognition System for Supporting Engineering Activities Downstream Conceptual Design. PhD thesis, New South Wale University (2007)

[10]   Joshi, S., Chang, T.C.: Graph-based Heuristics for Recognition of Machined Features from a 3D Solid Model. Computer-Aided Design 20(2), 58–66 (1988)

[11]   Ding, L., Yue, Y.: Novel ANN-based Feature Recognition Incorporating Design by Features. Computers In Industry 55, 197–222 (2004)

[12]   Ozturk, N., Ozturk, F.: Neural Network Based Non-Standard Feature Recognition to Integrate CAD and CAM. Computers in Industry 45, 123–135 (2001)

[13]   Dimov, S.S., Brousseau, E.B., Setchi, R.: A Hybrid Method for Feature Recognition in Computer-Aided Design Models. Journal of Engineering Manufacture 221, 79–96 (2007)

[14]   Liebowitz, J.: Knowledge Management and its Link to Artificial Intelligence. Expert Systems with Applications 20, 1–6 (2001)

[15]   Kerr, R.: Knowledge-based Manufacturing Management, pp. 126–177, 365 – 369. Addison-Wesley Press (1991)

[16]   Sowa, J.F. (ed.): Principles of Semantic Networks: Explorations in the Representation of Knowledge, pp. 13–41. Morgan Kaufmann Publishers (1991)

[17]   Zhang, H.L., Van der Velden, C.: Utilizing Knowledge Based Mechanisms in Automated Feature Recognition Processes. In: Hu, B., Liu, J., Chen, L., Zhong, N. (eds.) BI 2011. LNCS, vol. 6889, pp. 316–326. Springer, Heidelberg (2011)

Challenges and Opportunities for Health Information Systems Research

David Hansen

Australian E-Health Research Centre

Health systems around the world are increasing the adoption of electronic health records to improve access to patient data for administrative, treatment and research purposes.

The complexity of the data which is being stored in these electronic health records is providing a number of challenges for health information systems.

These challenges cover the capture of standardised data in an individual health information system, extracting necessary information from medical narratives, through to the processing of complex data including physiological, biomedical imaging and genomic data. However the largest challenges are in the interchange of the data and having health information systems use the data to provide intelligent decision support.

The transformation to a truly knowledge based healthcare system will require health information systems research provide solutions for these challenges. This talk will describe some of these challenges and give an overview to some current research topics and research which is now being adopted in health information systems.

J. He et al. (Eds.): HIS 2012, LNCS 7231, p. 60, 2012.

E-health in Australia – A General Practitioner's Perspective

Stanley Chiang

TLC Medical PTY LTD, Australia

Electronic Health, or E-health, has become a rather hot topic for quite a while now in Australia. The actual practice of it, however, has not been as quick as people would have hoped. There are a number of obstacles in its wider implementation, especially for general practitioners in the urban area.

This presentation will try to give an overview of the E-health in Australia, its current practice especially from a general practitioner's (GP) point of view. The advantages as well as its limitations will also be discussed, together with a forecasted future prospect of E-health in Australia.

J. He et al. (Eds.): HIS 2012, LNCS 7231, p. 61, 2012.
© Springer-Verlag Berlin Heidelberg 2012

Medical Devices: Panel Discussion

Terry Young

Brunel University, United Kingdom
Terry.Young@brunel.ac.uk

Most technology is developed along commercial lines and the development process is well understood in terms of capturing requirements, specifications, product or system engineering and marketing, logistics and sales. Medical technology, on the other hand, has the added burden of proving itself fit for purpose in the more highly regulated world of care delivery, where safety and performance are measured by those paying for the technology, often in quite different ways from the way in which standard business decisions are evaluated. In most parts of the world, the patient is not the only person paying – indeed, the patient may not pay at all – and so governments or insurers make purchasing decisions using their own concepts of value that may reflect the users' needs as a cohort, rather than a user's needs as an individual.

However such decisions are mediated, the situation when it comes to medical technologies is stringent on two fronts: the commercial and the clinical. Unless these perspectives, along with that of the end user can be unified in some way, one runs the risks that commercially viable products will fail, for instance, because medical services will not choose to use them, or because end users discard them and fail to comply by using them as intended. Clearly there are other risks – for instance that clinically useful products are never produced cheaply enough. So long as these fields – the commercial decisions to invest in, and develop a product or service, the clinical decisions around uptake and use, and the user response in terms of adopting the technology – remain isolated from one another, medical technology will always represent a risky proposition for both vendors and purchasers.

The MATCH project has spent the last 8 years researching common measures that can be applied from early in the development cycle to ensure the commercial viability, the value to healthcare systems, and the usefulness to users from the start. It is part of a new wave of research in health that applies economics, business process, and social science methods to reject failing ideas much earlier in the development cycle and to promote better ideas for investment, development, regulatory approval and sales in the marketplace.

The idea of a currency of value, shared as a concept by manufacturers, healthcare service providers and individual patients, has the potential to transform the way medical devices are developed and the impact they have upon healthcare.

This session aims to present different perspectives and to explore the potential impact of a more integrated view of value.

J. He et al. (Eds.): HIS 2012, LNCS 7231, p. 62, 2012.
© Springer-Verlag Berlin Heidelberg 2012

Color Image Sharing Method Based on Lagrange's Interpolating Polynomial

Guiqiang Chen[1], Jianjun Liu[1], and Liqin Wang[2]

[1] Institute of Information Science and Engineering, Hebei North University, Zhangjiakou, China
guiqiangchen@yahoo.com.cn, assemble8086@126.com
[2] Department of Electrical Engineering, Zhangjiakou Vocational College of Technology, Zhangjiakou, China

Abstract. In order to solve the problem of security during transmission of the large secret true color image, It is proposed that the secret image sharing method based on the Lagrange's interpolating polynomial, the n shadow images of the secret image were made by compressiong, substitute, encoding and disassemble to the secret image, each shadow image is hidden in an ordinary image so as not to attract an attacker's attention, the size of each stego image (in which a shadow image is hidden) is about 1/t of the secret image. Any t images in the n stego images can be used to recover the original secret image. The sharing principle and the recovery fomula are brought, the speed of the image sharing and recovery is heightened in this way, and the process of calculation is simplified. The method is discussed in different Galois domain, drawn the conditions that image block should satisfy, the best way to control the ratio of data expansion effectively and the relationships between security and anti-destructive. If the image as a mass of data, the method can be applied to the secure transmission and storage of huge amounts of data in the cloud computing.

Keywords: Lagrange's interpolating polynomial, secret image, stego image, image sharing.

1   Introduction

With the rapid development of Internet technology and the multimedia technology, the image that is difficult to store and transmit appears more and more on the computer screen, people are increasingly depend on the image, thus, the security issues of image became very prominent. Image sharing is an important theory part of information security, but also one of the main methods of image information hiding. Naor and Shamir proposed a VC[1] (Visual Cryptography) concept. Later, the VC scheme based on gray[2] and color images[3] have been constructed. Although the VC has some advantages, but because of the limited conditions of VC itself, the visual effects of the image recovered from sharing point has a wide gap between the original images. Therefore, in some occasion that high image quality requirement, VC is not as useful. Chang and Lin[4-6] proposed a scheme for sharing color image by (t, n) threshold, Lukac and Plataniotis[7] proposed a color secret image sharing scheme,

J. He et al. (Eds.): HIS 2012, LNCS 7231, pp. 63–75, 2012.

Although the recovered image can be as same effective as original image, However, because its use of (2,2) VC program ideas, Therefore, the secret sub-image generated by this way is as large as four times to the original size. Lvchao[8] proposed a image secret sharing scheme can ensure the recovered image quality, even can achieve the same quality as the original image, and the size of the secret sub-image is same to original image. But it does not hide the shadow image, one can find there are secret in it, and will attack and destroy it, therefore, the security is decreased. Even by hiding, the stego image will become too large because of the shadow image's size. Rey M.D.[9] proposed a relatively fast image secret sharing scheme based on simple binary matrix operations at Iberoamerican Congress on Pattern Recognition, 2008. But the scheme is demonstrated insecure by Esam Elsheh and A. Ben Hamza[10] , in [10], it is shown that care should be taken when choosing the matrices that corresponding to the shares, in particular if the rank of these singular matricesis not low enough then one can recover the secret image from only oneshare. This paper studies how a large true color secret image sharing to n pieces of color image that the size is 1/t to the original image, once get t pieces of shared color image, the true color secret image can be recoved. Thus, the problem of the secure transmission for large true color image is solved, And the n pieces of small stego sub-images is easy to transmit and not so easy to be found, to avoid be Suspected, attacked and destroied, even if n-t pieces of stego image are attacked, destroied or lost, the original secret image can be recovered security from the remaining t pieces of the stego image. The sharing storage theory and the directly recovery formula is presented in this paper, the speed of sharing and recover is improved, and the calculation process is simplified with the theory and the formula. At the same time, the method is discussed in different Galois domain, drawn the conditions that image block should satisfy, the best way to control the data rate of expansion effectively and the relationships between security and anti-destructive. If the image as a mass of data, the method can be applied to the secure transmission and storage of huge amounts of data in the cloud computing.

2   Theory of Image Sharing

2.1   Theory of Image Sharing and Recovery Based on Lagrange Interpolation Polynomial

Theory of Sharing
First define a bivariate one-way function $g(r,s)$, has the following properties: (1) Known r and s, is easy to calculate $g(r,s)$; (2) Known $g(r,s)$ and s, it is not feasible in the calculation to calculate r; (3) In the case of s unknown, for any r, it is difficult to calculate $g(r,s)$; (4) Known s, to find $r_1 \neq r_2$ satisfies $g(r_1,s) = g(r_2,s)$ is not feasible in the calculation; (5) Known r and $g(r,s)$, it is not feasible in the calculation to find s; (6) Known as many pair of the $(r_i, g(r_i,s))$, to find $g(r',s)$ is not feasible in the calculation, in which $r' \neq r_i$.

Assume $GF(q)$ is a finite field, where q is a large prime number, the sharing system working in $GF(q)$. Using the pixel values (or compression value) of t pieces of secret images to construct a polynomial in one unknown that the max power is t-1:

$$y = f(x) = (a_0 + a_1 x + a_2 x^2 + \cdots + a_{t-1} x^{t-1}) \bmod q \tag{1}$$

Where n ($n \geq t$) is the number of stego image that participate sharing storage. Every stego image that participate sharing storage corresponding a point (x_i, y_i), $1 \leq i \leq n$ on the curve determined by polynomial in one unknown $f(x)$, $y_i = f(x_i)$ is called value of shadow image, where x_i must be different from each other and should be keep secretly as a key, to improve security, the key is generated by polynomial in two unknown $g(r, s)$, it mesans $g(r_i, s_i) = x_i$, where r_i, s_i, x_i is in finite field $GF(q)$, r_i is the i-th stego image, s_i, a random integer selected by image sender is the shadow of key x_i, and is passed through a secret way to the image receiver. y_i can be published or embedded in original image r_i, the original stego image become a visual stego image with shadow image.

Theory of Recovery
When the image receiver calculate the pixel values (or compression value) $a_0, a_1, a_2, \cdots, a_{t-1}$ with any t ($t \leq n$) pieces of visual stego images which embedded shadow, the key x_i should be generated firstly with r_i, s_i and $g(r_i, s_i)$, secondly, drawn y_i from x_i to construct (x_i, y_i), t pieces of data (x_{k_i}, y_{k_i}) can be composed by any t ($t \leq n$), where $1 \leq k_i \leq n$, $i = 1, 2, \cdots, t$. A linear equations obtained by put the t pieces of data (x_{k_i}, y_{k_i}) into equation (1), obviously, the linear equations about $a_0, a_1, \cdots, a_{t-1}$ has unique solution when $x_{k_1}, x_{k_2}, \cdots, x_{k_t}$ different each other. This linear equations can be solved by general method, can also use the Lagrange interpolation polynomial and t piece of (x_{k_i}, y_{k_i}) to mke a polynomial in one unknown with t-1 power:

$$y = f(x) = \sum_{i=1}^{t} y_{k_i} \prod_{j=1, j \neq i}^{t} \frac{x - x_{k_j}}{x_{k_i} - x_{k_j}} \bmod q = (a_0 + a_1 x + a_2 x^2 + \cdots + a_{t-1} x^{t-1}) \bmod q \tag{2}$$

Expand the formula and calculate the coefficients of every term, the coefficients $a_0, a_1, \cdots, a_{t-1}$ is the pixel value of secret image, a coefficient can be expressed as:

$$a_{t-r} = (-1)^{r-1} \sum_{i=1}^{t} y_{k_i} \frac{A_{t-r}^i}{W_i} = (-1)^{r-1} \sum_{i=1}^{t} y_{k_i} \frac{A_{t-r}^i(k_1, k_2, \cdots, k_{i-1}, k_{i+1}, \cdots, k_t)}{\prod_{1 \leq i \neq j \leq t} (x_{k_i} - x_{k_j})} \bmod q \tag{3}$$

In equation (3), $W_i = \prod_{1 \leq j \neq i \leq t} (x_{k_i} - x_{k_j})$, and $A_{t-r}^i = A_{t-r}^i(k_1, k_2, \cdots, k_{i-1}, k_{i+1}, \cdots, k_t)$ has properties as following:

$$A_{t-1}^i(k_1, k_2, \cdots, k_{i-1}, k_{i+1}, \cdots, k_t) = 1$$

$$A_{t-2}^i(k_1, k_2, \cdots, k_{i-1}, k_{i+1}, \cdots, k_t) = x_{k_1} + x_{k_2} + \ldots + x_{k_{i-1}} + x_{k_{i+1}} + \ldots + x_{k_t}$$

$$A_{t-r}^i(k_1, k_2, \cdots, k_{i-1}, k_{i+1}, \cdots, k_t) = \sum_{(w_1, w_2, \ldots, w_{r-1}) \in Q} x_{w_1} x_{w_2} \ldots x_{w_{r-1}}$$

$$Q = \left\{ (w_1, w_2, \cdots, w_{r-1}) \middle| w_s \in \{k_1, k_2, \cdots, k_{i-1}, k_{i+1}, \cdots, k_t\}, 1 \le s \le r-1 \right\}$$

$$A_0^i(k_1, k_2, \cdots, k_{i-1}, k_{i+1}, \cdots, k_t) = x_{k_1} x_{k_2} \ldots x_{k_{i-1}} x_{k_{i+1}} \ldots x_{k_t}$$

In fact, it's easy to get the formula to calculate $a_0, a_1, \cdots a_{t-2}, a_{t-1}$, it is:

$$a_0 = \sum_{i=1}^t y_{k_i} \frac{(-1)^{t-1} \prod_{1 \le j \ne i \le t} x_{k_j}}{\prod_{1 \le j \ne i \le t} (x_{k_i} - x_{k_j})} \bmod q = f(0)$$

$$a_1 = \sum_{i=1}^t y_{k_i} \frac{(-1)^{t-2} \sum_{\substack{1 \le j \ne i \le t}} \prod_{\substack{1 \le v \le t \\ v \ne i, v \ne j}} x_{k_v}}{\prod_{1 \le j \ne i \le t} (x_{k_i} - x_{k_j})} \bmod q$$

$$a_{t-2} = \sum_{i=1}^t y_{k_i} \frac{-\sum_{1 \le j \ne i \le t} x_{k_j}}{\prod_{1 \le j \ne i \le t} (x_{k_i} - x_{k_j})} \bmod q$$

$$a_{t-1} = \sum_{i=1}^t y_{k_i} \frac{1}{\prod_{1 \le j \ne i \le t} (x_{k_i} - x_{k_j})} \bmod q \tag{4}$$

But if want to calculate a normal a_{t-r}, $A_{t-r}^i(k_1, k_2, \cdots, k_{i-1}, k_{i+1}, \cdots, k_t)$ should be calculated first, the calculation step is:

Assume $z_u = \begin{cases} x_{k_u}, 1 \le u \le i-1 \\ x_{k_{u+1}}, i \le u \le t-1 \end{cases}$

$$f_s(z) = \prod_{i=1}^s (z + z_i) = c_0 + c_1 z + \ldots + c_s z^s$$

Initialization: $s=1$, $c_0 = z_1$, $c_1 = 1$.

Recursive process: $s = s+1$, if $s < t$, then $c_0 = c_0 z_s$, $c_i = c_i z_s + c_{i-1} (0 < i < s)$, $c_s = 1$.

Termination: $s = t - 1, A_{t-r}^i (k_1, k_2, \cdots, k_{i-1}, k_{i+1}, \cdots, k_t) = c_{(t-r)} (0 < r \leq t)$ Get $a_0, a_1, \cdots, a_{t-1}$ by above steps, the pixel values $a_0, a_1, \cdots, a_{t-1}$ of t piece of secret image can ben recovered together.

2.2 Steps of Image Sharing and Recovery

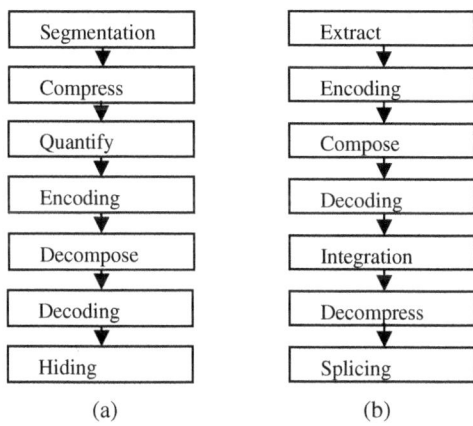

(a)   (b)

Fig. 1. Steps of image sharing (a) and recovery (b)

3 Algorithm for Image Sharing

In this experiment, the large prime numbers q is 17, t is 3, n is 5, Static 24 true color large original secret image is lena.bmp (120×120), see as Fig. 2 (a).

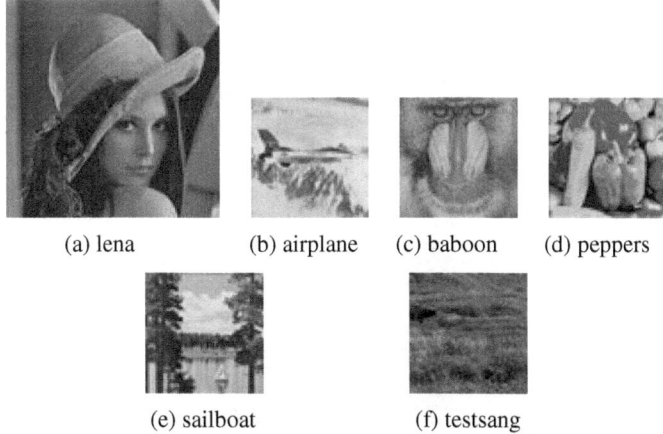

(a) lena   (b) airplane   (c) baboon   (d) peppers

(e) sailboat   (f) testsang

Fig. 2. Original secret image(120×120)-(a)and original stego image(60×60) (b), (c), (d), (e)

3.1   Image Segmentation and Splicing

Image segmentation means to express the large secret image with three component of R, G and B, Then each component been segmented to 8×8 image block, the image is carved into 15×15×3=675 blocks. Image splice is to compose 8×8 image blocks to R, G and B component and recovered the secret image, see as Fig. 3 (f).

3.2   Image Compression and Decompression

Image compression is Discrete Cosine Transform (DCT), Decompression is the inverse (IDCT). Firstly, every pixel value in 8×8 image blocks divided by 255, then get DCT coefficient matrix through forward Discrete Cosine Transform, IDCT process is the inverse DCT to DCT coefficient matrix.

3.3   Quantify and Integrate

Quantization process is to layout DCT coefficient matrix accordance with Z-shaped, Just take the top eleven coefficient (1 DC coefficient and 10 low frequency AC coefficient) to Quantify, Experiments show that the coefficient after eleven is very close to zero, they are ignored. Qualitify a 8×8 matrix of DCT coefficient into a 136 bit data stream, Compression ratio is 1/4, Compression ratio is near to 1/10 when JPEG algorithm be used. Quantification conversed the original secret image to 675×136=93825 bit stream. The integrate process is a reverse process of quatify.

3.4   Encoding and Decoding

Coding process is re-scheduling quantized 93825 bit stream to decimal digits from 0 to 16, using unequal-length coding, Experiment generated 20850 decimal digits, a decimal digit denote 4.5 bit. Decoding process is the reverse process of encoding.

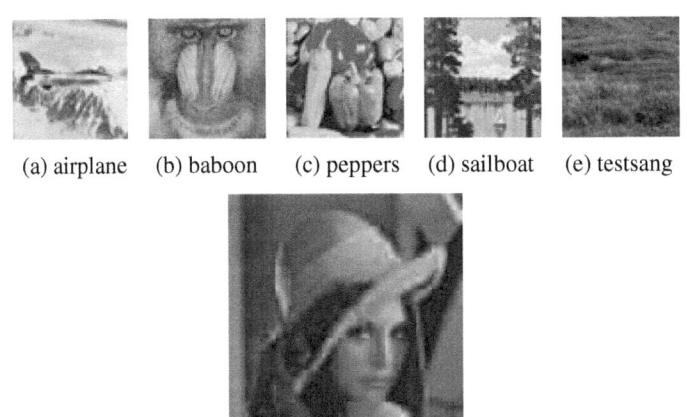

(a) airplane   (b) baboon   (c) peppers   (d) sailboat   (e) testsang

(f) lena

Fig. 3. Stego image with embeded secret (60×60)-(a), (b), (c), (d), (e) and recovered image from any 3 stego

3.5 Decomposition and Integration

Decomposition process just as stated as above, 20850 decimal digits which generated during encoding is divide into m=6950 group, each group j consists of t=3 decimal digits like $a_{j,0}, a_{j,1}, a_{j,2}$, a quadratic polynomial in one unknown obtained: $f_j(x) = (a_{j,0} + a_{j,1}x + a_{j,2}x^2) \bmod 17$ ($1 \le j \le 6950$). If the original BMP format images is like Fig. 2 (b),(c),(d),(e),(f), suppose the key $x_1 = 1$, $x_2 = 1$, $x_3 = 1$, $x_4 = 1$, $x_5 = 1$ are generated by one-way function $g(r,s)$, take them into $f_j(x)$, calculate the shadow image value $y_{j,1} = f_j(x_1) = f_j(1)$, the resul of decoding $y_{j,1}$ is 31275 bit stream, hide the bit stream into the image as Fig. 2(b). Similarly with the other, each group of decimal digit is calculated and hiden in stego image among Fig. 2(c), (d), (e), (f). Integration process is a reverse process to decomposition, iamge reciever can take any 3($3 \le 5$) piece of stego image from Fig. 3 (a),(b),(c),(d),(e), which is embeded shadow iamge, suppose as baboon, peppers and testsang. Firstly, the correspoding keys $x_2 = 2$, $x_3 = 3$, $x_5 = 5$ shoud be generated from one-way funcion $g(r,s)$, secondly, darwn the bit stream from corresponding stego image, decode it to $y_{j,2}, y_{j,3}, y_{j,5}$, thus, 3 pairs of data (x_2 , $y_{j,2}$),(x_3 , $y_{j,3}$),(x_5 , $y_{j,5}$) obtained, the coefficients $(a_{j,0}, a_{j,1}, a_{j,2})$ (where $1 \le j \le 6950$)to the quadratic polynomial in one unknown can be recovred from the formula (4), to get the data stream from 0 to 16, it is 20850 decimal digits.

3.6 Hiding and Extract

Stego imges is static 24 true color BMP format image in this experiment, consider the visula impact of R, G and B, take 2 bit of R component, 3 bit of G component and 4 bit of B component as redundant space to save secret data. Each stego image has 60×60×9=32400 bit redundant space to save 31275 bit stream from decoding. Extract process is a reverse process of hiding.

3.7 Result of Experiment

As shown in table 1, the objective evaluation is: the PSNR of recovered image is lower, the main reason is compression to image, has nothing to do with sharing, the PSNR can be increased by improving the compression algorithm. View from the subjective evaluation, the quality score of recovered image is 4, quality scale is good, prevent scale is that changes in image quality can be seen, but without prejudice to view. The quality score of stego image with secret data is 5, quality scale is better, prevent scale is that no deterioration in image quality can be seen.

Table 1. PSNR of the recovered image and the stego image with Embedded secret

	Recovered secret image(f)	Stego image with secret				
		a	b	c	d	e
PSNR	28.83	32.45	32.23	32.28	32.61	32.54

4   Comparison of Non-destructive Image Sharing in Different Galois Domain

For comparison, in Galois domain, suppose n of (t,n) threshold is 5, means n partici-pants or images privided by them, t=3 means t paritcipants can recover secret image. The original image is shown as Fig. 4(a), the resolution is (60×60), density resolution is 2^8, expressed as $F(i, j) = 2^b$ (where $1 \leq i$, $j \leq 60$, $b = 8$).

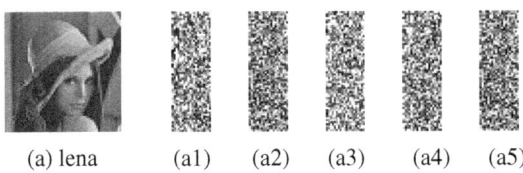

(a) lena   (a1)   (a2)   (a3)   (a4)   (a5)

Fig. 4. Original secret image (60×60)-(a)and shadow images (60×20) (a1), (a2), (a3), (a4), (a5)

4.1   Suppose Large Prime Number Is 17

For original image (lena.bmp) $F(i, j) = 2^b$ (where $1 \leq i$, $j \leq 60$, $b = 8$), seprate each pixel component into high 4 bit and low 4 bit, expressed as $FR(i, j) = 2^b$ (where $1 \leq i \leq 60$, $1 \leq j \leq 120$, $b = 4$). Every 3 decimal digit in $FR(i, j) = 2^b$ (where $1 \leq i \leq 60$, $1 \leq j \leq 120$, $b = 4$) take as a group like $a_{k,0}, a_{k,1}, a_{k,2}$ (where $a_{k,0} = F_R(i, l-1)$ $a_{k,1} = F_R(i, l)$ $a_{k,2} = F_R(i, l+1)$, ($1 \leq k \leq 2400$, $1 \leq i \leq 60$, $l = 3 \times e - 1$, $1 \leq e \leq 40$)). Construct a quadratic polynomial in one unkown $f_k(x) = (a_{k,0} + a_{k,1}x + a_{k,2}x^2) \bmod 17$ (where $1 \leq k \leq 2400$) with $a_{k,0}, a_{k,1}, a_{k,2}$ as coef-ficient. The 5 keys to 5 participants is $x_1 = 1, x_1 = 2, x_1 = 3, x_1 = 4, x_1 = 5$, take them into $f_k(x)$ respectively, calsulate the shadow value $y_{k,1} = f_k(x_1) = f_k(1)$, $y_{k,2} = f_k(x_2) = f_k(2)$, $y_{k,3} = f_k(x_3) = f_k(3)$, $y_{k,4} = f_k(x_4) = f_k(4)$, $y_{k,5} = f_k(x_5) = f_k(5)$ (where $1 \leq k \leq 2400$). Decode the $y_{k,1}$ (it is a decimal digit from 0 to 16) to shadow bit stream and hide the bit stream into stego image provided by r1. The other is similarly to it. In order to facilitate comparison, encoding the $y_{k,1}$ to 5 bit binary digit, $y_{k,1}$ is combined to a pixel, the combined image is a shadow image $F_1(i, j) = 2^b$ (where $1 \leq i \leq 60$, $1 \leq j \leq 20$, $b = 10$) shown as Fig. 4(a1). The others is similarly to it and shown as Fig. 4(a2),(a3),(a4),(a5).

When the secret image to be recovered, any 3 participants can draw shadow bit stream from stego image with shadow, and encoding the bit stream into y_{k,w_j} ($1 \leq k \leq 2400$, $1 \leq w_j \leq 5$, $1 \leq j \leq 3$), generated the key x_{w_j} by one-way func-tion $g(r,s)$, construct data pair of (x_{w_j} , y_{k,w_j}) (where $1 \leq k \leq 2400$, $1 \leq w_j \leq 5$, $1 \leq j \leq 3$), $a_{k,i}$ ($1 \leq k \leq 2400$, $1 \leq j \leq 3$)can be calculated from formula (4), and

$F_R(i,l-1) = a_{k,1}$, $F_R(i,l) = a_{k,2}$, $F_R(i,l+1) = a_{k,3}$ ($1 \leq k \leq 2400$, $1 \leq i \leq 60$, $l = 3 \times e - 1, 1 \leq e \leq 40$) is recovered image. If the stego image is damaged or there is noise in it, the recovered image will lose some information, shown as Fig. 5. The solution is find the pixel positions which are damaged or noised, then take use of the correspoding pixel in other stego image that is non-deteioration to recover.

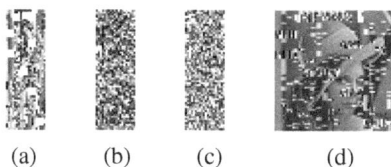

(a)   (b)   (c)   (d)

Fig. 5. Shadow images contains noise (a), (b), (c) and recovered secret image (d)

4.2   Suppose Large Prime Number Is 257

For original image (lena.bmp) $F(i,j) = 2b$ (where $1 \leq i$, $j \leq 60$, $b = 8$), each rows of pixel as a group, expressed as $a_{k,0}, a_{k,1}, \cdots, a_{k,v}$ (where $a_{k,v} = F(i,j)$ ($1 \leq k \leq 60$, $0 \leq v \leq 59$, $1 \leq i \leq 60$, $1 \leq j \leq 60$)). Construct a 59 power polynomial in one unkown $f_k(x) = (a_{k,0} + a_{k,1}x + \cdots + a_{k,v}x^v) \mod 257$ (where $1 \leq k \leq 60$, $0 \leq v \leq 59$). Dvide the Galois domain $GF(257)$ (ie 0 to 256) into 5 integer domain $GF(1 \leq n \leq 5)$, the 5 integer domain $GF_1(1 \sim 50)$, $GF_2(51 \sim 100)$, $GF_3(101 \sim 150)$, $GF_4(151 \sim 200)$ and $GF_5(201 \sim 256)$ are correspoding to 5 participants, each participant take any 20 integers different from each other from their integer domain as the key $x_{n,j}$ (where $1 \leq n \leq 5$, $1 \leq j \leq 20$), take the 20 integers into $f_k(x)$ and get the shadow value $y_{k,n,j} = f_k(x_{n,j})$ (where $1 \leq k \leq 60$, $1 \leq n \leq 5$, $1 \leq j \leq 20$). Decode $y_{k,n,j}$ (ie 0 to 256) to shadow bit stream and hide it into the stego image provided by participant r_n. In order to facilitate comparison, encoding the $y_{k,1}$ to 9 bit binary digit as a pixel, the shadow image $F_1(i,n,j) = 2^b$ (where $1 \leq i \leq 60$, $1 \leq n \leq 5$, $1 \leq j \leq 20$, $b = 9$) obtained. Shown as Fig. 6.

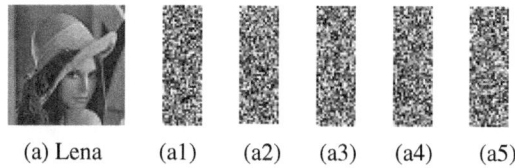

(a) Lena   (a1)   (a2)   (a3)   (a4)   (a5)

Fig. 6. Original secret image (a) and shadow images (a1), (a2), (a3), (a4), (a5)

When the secret image to be recovered, any 3 participants can draw shadow bit stream from stego image with shadow, and encoding the bit stream into $y_{k,n_w,j}$ ($1 \leq k \leq 60$, $1 \leq n_w \leq 5$, $1 \leq w \leq 3$), construct data pair of $(x_{n_w,j}, y_{k,n_w,j})$ (where

$1 \leq k \leq 60$, $1 \leq n_w \leq 5$, $1 \leq w \leq 3$, $1 \leq j \leq 20$)with the key x_{w_j} $x_{n_w,j}$ (where $1 \leq n_w \leq 5$, $1 \leq w \leq 3$, $1 \leq j \leq 20$), $a_{k,v}$ ($1 \leq k \leq 60$, $0 \leq v \leq 59$) can be calculated from formula (4), and $F(i, j) = a_{k,v}$ ($1 \leq k \leq 60$, $0 \leq v \leq 59$, $1 \leq i \leq 60$, $1 \leq j \leq 60$) is recovered image. If the stego image is damaged or there is noise in it, the recovered image will lose some information, shown as Fig. 7. The solution is find the rows positions which are damaged or noised, then take use of the correspoding rows in other stego image that is non-deteioration to recover.

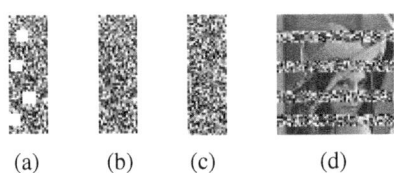

(a)   (b)   (c)   (d)

Fig. 7. Shadow images contain noise (a),(b),(c) and recovered image (d)

4.3   Suppose Large Prime Number Is 65287

For original image (lena.bmp) $F(i, j) = 2^b$ (where $1 \leq i$, $j \leq 60$, $b = 8$), each rows of pixel as a group, expressed as $a_0, a_1, \cdots, a_k$ (where $a_k = F(i, j) * 256 + F(i, j+1)$, $1 \leq j \leq 60$). Construct a 1799 power polynomial in one unkown $f(x) = (a_0 + a_1 x + \cdots + a_k x^k) \bmod 65287$ (where $0 \leq k \leq 1799$). Dvide the Galois domain $GF(65287)$ (ie 0 to 65286) into 5 integer domain $GF(1 \leq n \leq 5)$, the 5 integer domain $GF_1(1 \sim 13000)$, $GF_2(13001 \sim 26000)$, $GF_3(26001 \sim 39000)$, $GF_4(39001 \sim 52000)$ and $GF_5(52001 \sim 65286)$ are correspoding to 5 participants, each participant take any 600 integers different from each other from their integer domain as the key $x_{n,j}$ (where $1 \leq n \leq 5$, $1 \leq j \leq 600$), take the 600 integers into $f_k(x)$ and get the shadow value $y_{n,j} = f(x_{n,j})$ (where $1 \leq n \leq 5$, $1 \leq j \leq 600$). Decode $y_{k,n,j}$ (ie 0 to 65286) to shadow bit stream and hide it into the stego image provided by participant r_n, In order to facilitate comparison, encoding the $y_{k,1}$ to 16 bit binary digit as two 8 bit pixel, the shadow image $\hat{f}(n, i, j) = 2^b$ (where $1 \leq n \leq 5$, $1 \leq i \leq 60$, $1 \leq j \leq 20$, $b = 8$) obtained. Shown as Fig. 8.

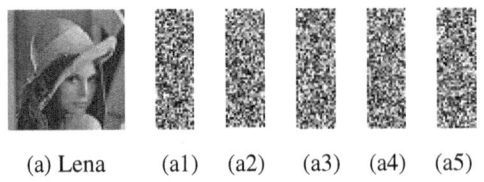

(a) Lena   (a1)   (a2)   (a3)   (a4)   (a5)

Fig. 8. Original secret image (60×60)-(lena) and shadow images(60×20) (a1), (a2), (a3), (a4), (a5)

When the secret image to be recovered, any 3 participants can draw shadow bit stream from stego image with shadow, and encoding the bit stream into $y_{n_w,j}$ ($1 \leq n_w \leq 5$, $1 \leq w \leq 3$, $1 \leq j \leq 600$), construct data pair of ($x_{n_w,j}$, $y_{k,n_w,j}$) with the private key $x_{n_w,j}$ (where $1 \leq n_w \leq 5$, $1 \leq w \leq 3$, $1 \leq j \leq 600$), a_k ($0 \leq k \leq 1799$) can be calculated from formula (4), and $F(i,j) = \left\lfloor \dfrac{a_k}{257} \right\rfloor$, $F(i,j+1) = a_k - 257 * \left\lfloor \dfrac{a_k}{257} \right\rfloor$ (where $0 \leq k \leq 1799$, $1 \leq i \leq 60$, $j = 2 \times s - 1$, $1 \leq s \leq 30$) is recovered image. If the stego image is damaged or there is noise in it, it impossible to recover the original secret image, shown as Fig. 9. The solution is to discard the shadow image which are damaged or noised, then take use of the correspoding shadow images provided by other stego image that is non-deteioration to recover.

(a)   (b)   (c)   (d)

Fig. 9. Shadow images contain noise (a), (b), (c) and recovered secret image (d)

4.4   Comparison of Three Cases

In three different Galois domains above, comparing the overall performance of iamge sharing about security, ratio of data expansion and anti-destructive, the best method on how to block the image better and how to control the ratio of data expansion effectively is presented.

If threshold is (t=3,n=5), For example, the original secret image is lena.bmp shown as Fig. 2(a), the resolution is (60×60), desity resolution is 28, non-destructive sharing, and encode in same length.

Table 2. Comparison of variety performance in different Galois field

GF(q)	17	257	65287
Pixel (bits)	4	8	16
block (pixel)	1.5	1 row	all
Power k	3	60	1800
Shadow pixel (bits)	5	9	17
Shadow pixel number (n)	5	100	3000
Repeat times (j)	2400	60	1
Private keys	1	20	600
Private key space	16/5	256/5	65286/5
Ratio of pixel bits expansion	1.25	1.125	1.0625
Ratio of pixel number expansion	5/3	5/3	5/3
security	low	medium	high
Anti-destructive	high	medium	low

Shown as table 2, the larger Galois field $GF(q)$, the more private keys. And the more private keys, the more security and the lower of anti-destructive. Original image must be blocked in Galois field $GF(q)$, the pixel bits less than q, the number of pixel in original image is an integer multiple of the number of pixel in each block image, so as to meet threshold theory better. The ratio of data expansion has two case, one is the ratio of pixel bits, using equal length coding, it is expressed as $\dfrac{pixel\ bits\ in\ shadow\ image}{pixel\ bits\ in\ original\ image}$, the larger Galois field $GF(q)$, the lower ratio of pixel bits, because of the max pixel bits in original image is old number and less than the max prime number q in Galois field, but the max pixel bits in shadow image is q-1, it must be a even number and great than pixel bits in original image, because of using equal length coding, shadow pixel bits is a bit more than original pixel bits, thus, the larger Galois field $GF(q)$, the lower ratio of pixel bits. The other is ratio of pixel number expansion, it is expressed as $\dfrac{pixel\ number\ in\ shadow\ image}{pixel\ number\ in\ original\ image} = \dfrac{n}{t}$, has no relationship with Galois field $GF(q)$, just has relationship with the threshold. So, the ratio of data expansion can be expressed as a product of pixel bits and pixel number, it can be controled by limit pixel bits and pixel number.

5   Conclusion

A lossy compression of image sharing scheme is presented in this paper, a large true colr secret image is shared into n pieces of coloe stego imge whose size is 1/t to the secret image. The original image can be recovered from any t pieces of stego image with secret; it will get no information if the stego imgae with secret is less than t, this scheme is more secure than the one in [9]. The innovation in this paper is presenting a recovery formula of coefficient, greatly enhance the recovery speed of the image, and simplify the calculation process. In practice, this sharing scheme saves storage space, reduces the transmission time, savs storage and transmission resources significantly, solved the security problem during transmission of large true color secret image, the secret image is easy to transmission and hard to be found after sharing, avoided been suspected, attacked and destoried, even if there are n-t pieces of stego image been damaged or lose, the original image can be recovered from the remained t pieces of stego image. By comparing the experiment results, obtained the conditions of image block should satisfied, the best way to control the ratio of data expansion effectively, and the relationship between security and anti-destructive.

References

1. Naor, M., Shamir, A.: Visual Cryptography. In: De Santis, A. (ed.) EUROCRYPT 1994. LNCS, vol. 950, pp. 1–12. Springer, Heidelberg (1995)
2. Blundo, C., De Santis, A., Naor, M.: Visual cryptography for grey level images. Information Processing Letters 75(6), 255–259 (2000)

3. Hou, Y.C.: Visual cryptography for color images. Pattern Recognition 36(7), 1619–1629 (2003)
4. Chang, C.C., Lin, I.C.: A New (t,n) Threshold Image Hiding Scheme for Sharing a Secret Color Image. In: Proceedings of the International Conference on Communication Technology, Beijing, vol. 1, pp. 196–202 (2003)
5. Chang, C.C., Chuang, J.C.: An image intellectual property protection scheme for gray level images using visual secret sharing strategy. Pattern Recognition Letters 23(8), 931–941 (2002)
6. Yang, C.C., Chang, T.Y., Hwang, M.S.: A (t,n) multi-secret sharing scheme. Applied Mathematics and Computations 151(2), 483–490 (2004)
7. Lukac, R., Plataniotis, K.N.: Color image secret sharing. Electronics Letters 40(9), 529–531 (2004)
8. Lvchao, Yu, M., Liu, Y.: The secret image sharing scheme based on Lagrange interpolation polynomial. Journal of Huazhong University of Science and Technology 33(12), 285–289 (2005)
9. del Rey, A.M.: A Matrix-Based Secret Sharing Scheme for Images. In: Ruiz-Shulcloper, J., Kropatsch, W.G. (eds.) CIARP 2008. LNCS, vol. 5197, pp. 635–642. Springer, Heidelberg (2008)
10. Elsheh, E., Ben Hamza, A.: Comments on Matrix-Based Secret Sharing Scheme for Images. In: Bloch, I., Cesar Jr., R.M. (eds.) CIARP 2010. LNCS, vol. 6419, pp. 169–175. Springer, Heidelberg (2010)

Automation in Cytomics: A Modern RDBMS Based Platform for Image Analysis and Management in High-Throughput Screening Experiments

E. Larios[1], Y. Zhang[2], K. Yan[1], Z. Di[3], S. LeDévédec[3],
F. Groffen[2], and F. J. Verbeek[1]

[1] Section Imaging and Bioinformatics, LIACS, Leiden University, Leiden, The Netherlands
{elarios,kyan,fverbeek}@liacs.nl
[2] Centrum Wiskunde and Informatica, Amsterdam, The Netherlands
{Ying.Zhang,Fabian.Groffen}@cwi.nl
[3] Department of Toxicology, LACDR, Leiden University, Leiden, The Netherlands
{z.di,s.e.ledevedec}@lacdr.leidenuniv.nl

Abstract. In cytomics bookkeeping of the data generated during lab experiments is crucial. The current approach in cytomics is to conduct High-Throughput Screening (HTS) experiments so that cells can be tested under many different experimental conditions. Given the large amount of different conditions and the readout of the conditions through images, it is clear that the HTS approach requires a proper data management system to reduce the time needed for experiments and the chance of man-made errors. As different types of data exist, the experimental conditions need to be linked to the images produced by the HTS experiments with their metadata and the results of further analysis. Moreover, HTS experiments never stand by themselves, as more experiments are lined up, the amount of data and computations needed to analyze these increases rapidly. To that end cytomic experiments call for automated and systematic solutions that provide convenient and robust features for scientists to manage and analyze their data. In this paper, we propose a platform for managing and analyzing HTS images resulting from cytomics screens taking the automated HTS workflow as a starting point. This platform seamlessly integrates the whole HTS workflow into a single system. The platform relies on a modern relational database system to store user data and process user requests, while providing a convenient web interface to end-users. By implementing this platform, the overall workload of HTS experiments, from experiment design to data analysis, is reduced significantly. Additionally, the platform provides the potential for data integration to accomplish genotype-to-phenotype modeling studies.

1 Introduction

Recent developments in microscopy technology allows various cell and structure phenotypes to be visualized using genetic engineering. With a time-lapse image-acquisition approach, dynamic activities such as cell migration can be captured and analyzed. When performed in large-scale via robotics, such approach is often referred to as a High-Throughput Screening (HTS). At the work floor this is often called "screen". In cytometry, HTS experiments, at both cellular and structural level, are widely employed

J. He et al. (Eds.): HIS 2012, LNCS 7231, pp. 76–87, 2012.

in functional analysis of chemical compounds, antibodies and genes. With automated image analysis, a quantification of cell activity can be extracted from HTS experiments. In this manner, biological hypothesis or diagnostic testing can be verified via machine learning using the results from the image analysis. HTS experiments, supported by automated image analysis and data analysis, can depict an objective understanding of the cell response to various treatments or exposures.

In this paper, we set our scope to the bioinformatics aspects of HTS. An HTS experiment starts with the design of a culture plate layout containing $N \times M$ wells in which the cells are kept, cultured and to which experimental conditions are applied. The response of the cells is then recorded through time-lapse (microscopy) imaging and the resulting time-lapse image sequence is the basis for the image analysis. The design of the plate layout is a repository of the experiment as a whole. From a study of the workflow of biologists, we have established an HTS workflow system.

Currently, spreadsheet applications are commonly used for bookkeeping the information generated during the workflow of HTS experiments. This approach has many drawbacks. It usually takes months to finish a complete experiment, i.e., from the plate design to the data analysis. Furthermore, images produced by the HTS experiments are not linked properly with their metadata and the analysis results. This scenario makes it difficult to do a proper knowledge discovery. So, most of the process within the workflow of HTS experiments are developed manually, which is highly prone to man made errors. Moreover, spreadsheets often differ in format and are not stored in a central place. This makes it hard for scientists from even the same institute to search, let alone to disclose their results in a uniform and efficient way.

To eventually tackle all these issues, we propose an *HTS platform* for managing and analysing cytomic images produced by HTS experiments. The platform seamlessly integrates the whole HTS workflow into a single system and provides end-users a convenient GUI to interact with the system. The platform consists of a layered architecture. First, an end-user layer that is responsible for the interaction with the scientists who perform different HTS experiments in cytomics. Then, the middleware layer that is responsible of the management of secure and reliable communication among the different components in the platform. Finally, a database-computational layer, in charge of the repository and execution of the image and data analysis.

Preliminary tests show that by using this platform, the overall workload of HTS experiments, from experiment design to data analysis, is reduced significantly. This is because, among others, in the HTS platform, the design of plate layout is done automatically. Using spreadsheets, it takes an experienced biologist one week to manually finish the mapping of 400-600 gene targets, while it takes less than a day to use the plate design modular in the HTS system. It also enables queries over datasets of multiple experiments. Thus, automation in cytomics provides a robust environment for HTS experiments.

To sum up, the contributions of this work include:

1. Establishing a workflow system of the HTS experiments (Section 2).
2. An integrated platform to automate data management and image analysis of cytomic HTS experiments (Section 3).

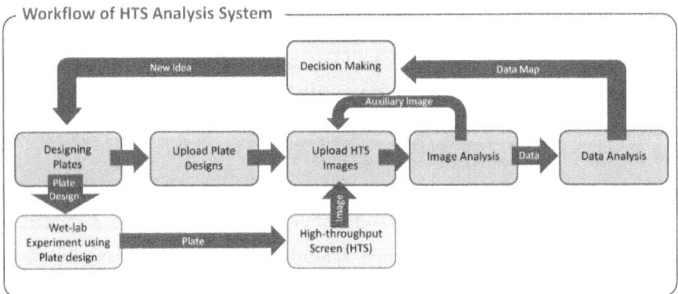

Fig. 1. Workflow of the HTS Analysis System

3. The design of the database to store (almost) all data produced and used in the HTS experiments (Section 4).

Finally, we discusses related work in Section 5 and conclude in Section 6.

2   Workflow of the HTS Experiments

A workflow of a general HTS experiment is shown in Figure 1, where the typical stages are depicted separately. In this section, we describe the four functional modules in this *HTS workflow*: (1) plate design, (2) image analysis, (3) data management, and (4) pattern recognition [13].

Plate Layout Design Module.   The design of a plate is considered as the cornerstone for an HTS experiment. Therefore, we have developed a Graphical User Interface (GUI) in our HTS platform to construct the layout for a plate (see Figure 2). The GUI allows end-users to rapidly deploy, modify and search through plate designs, to which auxiliary data such as experimental protocols, images, analysis result and supplementary literature is attached. In addition, the plate design provides a fast cross-reference mechanism in comparing data from various origins. This module is also used as the front end for the visualisation of results such as using heat maps, cell detection or motion trajectories.

Image Analysis Module.   In the acquisition phase, the time-lapse sequences are connected to the plate design. Customized image processing and analysis tools or algorithms are applied on the raw images to obtain features for each of the different treatments. Our image analysis kernel is deployed to provide a customised and robust image segmentation and object tracking algorithm [14], dedicated to various types of cytometry. The current package covers solutions to cell migration, cellular matrix dynamics and structure dynamics analysis (see Figures 3, 4, 5). The package has been practised in HTS experiments for toxic compound screening of cancer metastasis [8,11], wound-and-recovery of kidney cells [11] and cell matrix adhesion complex signaling, etc [4].

The segmentation of objects is conducted using our watershed masked clustering algorithm, an innovative algorithm dedicated to fluorescence microscopy imaging. Frequently, the efficiency of fluorescence staining or protein fusion is subjective and highly unpredictable, which results in disorganized intensity bias within and between cells

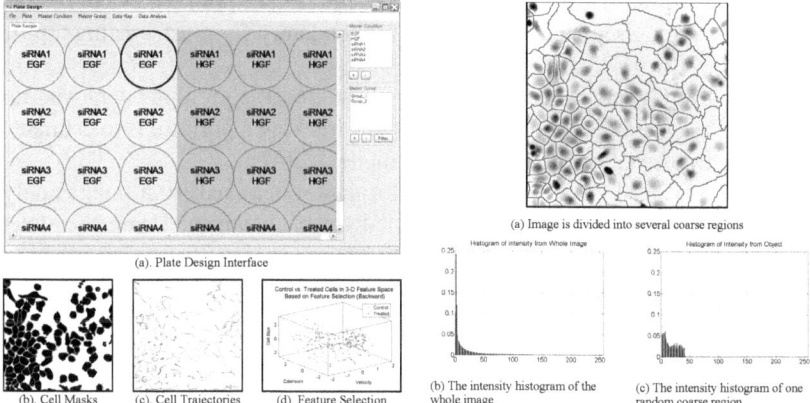

(a). Plate Design Interface

(b). Cell Masks   (c). Cell Trajectories   (d). Feature Selection

Fig. 2. Plate layout design GUI and visualisation of results, including cell masks, motion trajectories and machine learning conclusions

(a) Image is divided into several coarse regions

(b) The intensity histogram of the whole image

(c) The intensity histogram of one random coarse region

Fig. 3. Image and coarse regions

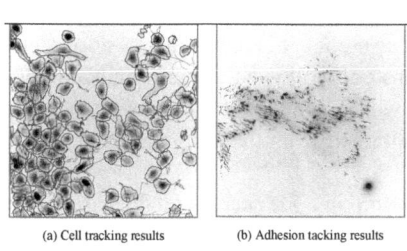

(a) Cell tracking results   (b) Adhesion tacking results

Fig. 4. Using our image analysis solution, the phenotypic measurements of (a) live cells and (b) adhesion can be extracted

Control vs. Treated Cells in 3-D Feature Space Based on Feature Selection (Backward)

Fig. 5. Phenotypic characterization of the Epidermal Growth Factor (EGF) treatment using a highly aggressive cancer cell line, the illustrated features are picked by branch-and-bound feature selection. The EGF-treated cell group shows a significant increased migration velocity.

(see Figure 3a). The principle behind our algorithm is to divide such an extreme and multimodal optimization problem (Figure 3b) into several sub-optimal yet uni-modal optimization problems (Figure 3c). Such divided-and-conquer strategy provides an extended flexibility in searching intensity thresholds in each image. Contrary to bottom-up segmentation strategies such as the Otsu algorithm, our solution prevents undertraining by introduce a flexible kernel definition based on the congenital (intensity) homogeneity of an image. Unlike top-down segmentation strategies such as the level-set algorithm, our current algorithm prevents overtraining by overlooking into the intensity distribution of the completely homogeneous region, therefore, less sensitive to local intensity distortion; in addition, our algorithm does not require any prior knowledge or manual interference during segmentation while it is mandatory for most existing top-down methods.

The tracking of objects is accomplished by customised algorithms deployed in the image analysis package. The principle behind this tracking algorithm is to estimate the minimum mean shift vector based on a given model [8,14].

With the binary masks and trajectories information obtained from image analysis, several phenotypic measurements are extracted for each object. Using the state-of-art pattern recognition and statistical analysis techniques, the effect of chemical compounds can be easily quantified and compared (Figure 5). Depending on the experiment setting, our package may employ up to 31 phenotypic measurements during the analysis.

The image analysis module is designed as a web service API module in the HTS platform. As the image analysis computation requires large image volumes to be processed, a high performance scientific computer cloud is used to obtain results in reasonable time.

Data Management Module. In cytomics bookkeeping of the information generated during lab experiments is crucial. The amount of image data can easily exceed the terabyte-scale. However, currently spreadsheets applications are commonly used for this purpose. The accessibility of large volume of image data already poses an obstacle in the current stage.

After scientists having performed HTS experiments, it is necessary to store meta information, incluing the experiment type, the protocol followed, experimental conditions used and the plate design, and associate each well in the plate to the raw images generated during the experiments and the results obtained from the image and data analysis when these processes are completed.

Currently, the large volume of images are stored in a file server and they are accessed following a standard naming convention. The locations of the files are stored in the spreadsheet application used for the experiment, but this is not suitable for knowledge discovery later on or querying the results obtained in the analysis process.

The platform uses MonetDB, a modern column-based database management system (DBMS) as a repository of the different types of data that are used in the HTS Workflow System. Each component of the architecture communicate with the database through web services (Figure 7). This makes the future integration with other APIs more flexible.

Data and Pattern Analysis Module. Typical to the kind of analysis required for cytomics data is that the temporal as well as the spatial dimension is included in the analysis. The spatial dimension tells us where a cell or cell structure is, whereas the time-point informs us when it is at that particular location. Features are derived from the images that are time lapse series (2D+T or 3D+T). Over these features pattern recognition procedures are multi-parametric analysis. It is a basic form of machine learning solution, which frequently employed in the decision-making procedure of biological and medical research. A certain pattern recognition procedure may be engaged in supporting various conclusions. For example, a clustering operation based on cell morphological measurements may provide an innate subpopulation within a cell culture [8] while a

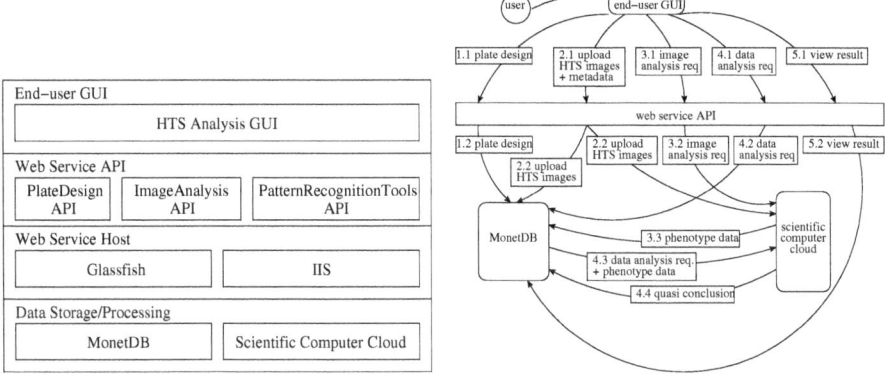

Fig. 6. The HTS analysis platform architecture   **Fig. 7.** Flow of control of the HTS platform

classification operation using temporal phenotypic profile can be used to identify of each cell phase during division [10]. The service that deals with the pattern recognition is based on the PR-Tools software package developed at the Delft University of Technology (www.prtools.org).

The PR-Tools library can be integrated in MatLab [9] and we have used it in that fashion. In order to deal with the temporal dimension, the package was extended with specific elements to allow temporal analysis over spatial data. The prototype data analysis module is implemented as a web service API based on output generated by MatLab deployment tools. The availability of MatLab with PR-Tools within this architecture allows for rapid prototyping with a range of complex mathematical algorithms. In addition, PR-Tools in MatLab has its own GUI and in this manner data mining strategies can be explored by the end-user without in-depth knowledge of machine learning. The flexibility that is accomplished in this manner is efficient for the end-users as well as the software engineers who need to maintain and implement the services for machine learning.

3   System Architecture of the HTS Analysis Platform

To automate the workflow of HTS experiments and provide the users with a convenient interface to interact with the system, we have designed an *HTS analysis platform* [13] (for short: HTS platform), which has a layered architecture. Figure 6 depicts the components in each layer of the architecture.

The GUI Layer. The HTS platform enables end-users to carry out complete HTS experiments using a single graphical user interface, i.e., the *HTS Analysis GUI*. This way, even for end-users without extensive knowledge in cytomics, it is easy to learn how to do HTS experiments in cytometry. In addition, data sets produced under different conditions or from different HTS experiments are available through one interface. This also counts for the resulting data from each step in an HTS experiment. As a result, end-users can easily view, compare and analyse the different data sets.

The Web Service Layers. The two lower layers together, through web services, support every step in the HTS workflow that is done on the computers, i.e., the middle most five boxes in Figure 1 (the other steps involves human actions). The APIs are grouped in three modules in the *Web Service API* layer, with each module corresponding to a module described in Section 2. This module structure allows quick development, error isolation and easy extending with more functional modules in the future.

We chose SOAP (Simple Object Access Protocol) messages for invoking the web services and receiving results, because of its approved interoperability in web applications and heterogeneous environments. In case of the HTS platform, we must support different programming languages. Using SOAP makes it possible for various languages to invoke operations from each other. Transportation of the data generated by an experiment is integrated into web service calls. Large files are transmitted as attachments of the SOAP messages. To do this, the MTOM (Message Transmission Optimization Mechanism) feature [6] of the Glassfish Server is used. Ensuring error free data transmission and controlling user access permissions are done at the application level.

The Data Storage/Processing Layer. There are two components in this layer. For the data management component, we made a conscious choice for MonetDB (www.monetdb.org), a modern column-based database system, after having considered different alternatives. For instance, in the initial design of the database schema, we have considered to use an XML supporting DBMS such as Oracle or Microsoft SQL Server in order to facilitate a flexible integration with other systems in the future. However, it is generally known that, compared with relational data, XML data requires considerable storage overhead and processing time, which makes it unsuitable as a storage format for the large volume of cytomic data. Moreover, traditional database systems are optimised for transactional queries, while in cytomics, we mainly have analytical queries. Traditional database systems generally carry too much overhead when processing analytical queries [2]. What we need is a database optimised for data mining applications. MonetDB is a leading open source database system that has been designed specially for such applications [2]. It has been well-known for its performance in processing analytical queries on large scale data [3]. Thus, in our final decision, we use SOAP messages (i.e., XML format) to exchange small sized (meta-)data, but use MonetDB to store a major portion of the data produced and used during the HTS experiments, including all metadata and binary data generated during analysis. Additionally, a powerful scientific computer cluster is used to store the raw image data resulting from microscopy and to execute computing intensive image analysis tools. However, the future plan is to move also the raw data and as much as possible operations on them into the database system.

Flow of Control. The diagram shown in Figure 7 illustrates the flows of the control in the HTS platform. How the main features of the platform are executed is shown by five sequences of annotated arrows starting from the end-user GUI. Arrows handling the same operation are grouped together by a major number, while the minor numbers corresponds to the order of a particular step that is called in its containing sequence. Below we describe each sequence.

Sequence 1 handles a new plate design, which is straightforward: the request is sent to MonetDB and a new entry is created. Sequence 2 handles uploading an HTS image request. Because currently the raw image data is stored separately, this request results in

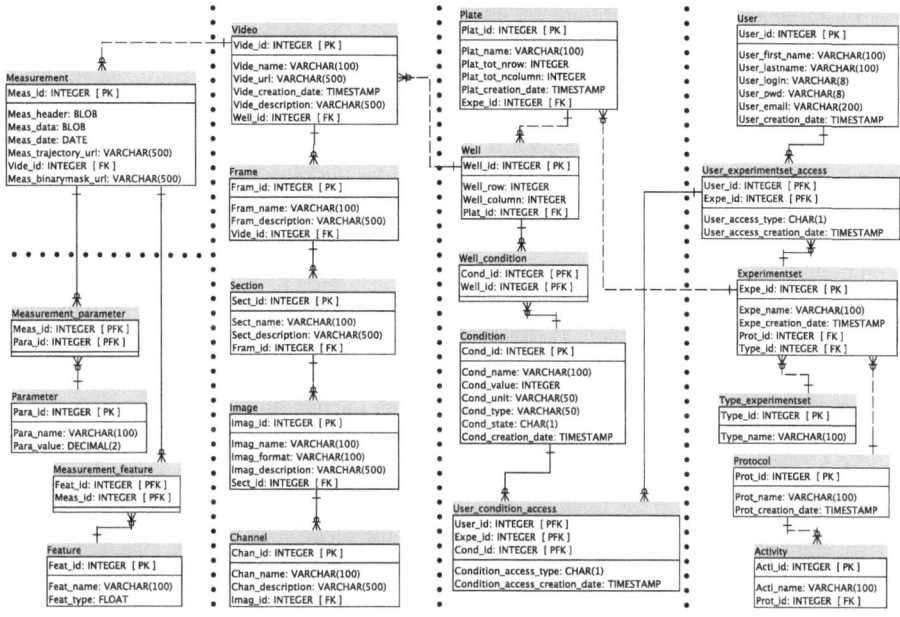

Fig. 8. The database schema used by the HTS platform

the metadata being stored in MonetDB while the binary data is stored on the scientific super computer. Sequence 3 handles an image analysis request, which is passed to the scientific super computer, since both the data to be analysed and the tools are there. Then the results are sent to MonetDB and stored there (step 3.3). Sequence 4 handles a data analysis request, which is first sent to MonetDB. Then, MonetDB passes both the request and the necessary data (obtained from the image analysis) to the scientific super computer for execution. The results are again stored in MonetDB. Since the most used data is stored at one place, in sequence 5, a view results request can be handled by just requesting data of both image analysis and data analysis from MonetDB. In the GUI, the results are displayed with the corresponding plate layout, as indicated in Figure 2.

Summary. In this section, we described the software architecture of the HTS platform, how its main features are processed, and how web services are used for the communication with the DBMS and the dedicated scientific computer cloud. In the next section, we present how all data is stored in the DBMS.

4   Database Design

The complete relational database schema designed to store the metadata, images and binary data generated during the execution of the HTS workflow is shown in Figure 8. The schema can be roughly divided into five regions (separated by the dotted lines): i) users and the experiment sets they work on, ii) the design of the culture plates, iii) raw images acquired during a single HTS experiment, iv) results of image analysis, and v) results of data analysis. Below we explain how the data is stored in each of these regions and the relationships among the tables.

Users and Experiment Sets. The basic information of a user is stored in the table User. Every user can start with a new ExperimentSet, who is then also the author of this set of experiments. All analyses in an experiment set are of the same Type (see also "*Raw Images*" below) and are carried out under the same Protocol, which in turn can have zero-or-more Activity attached to it. A protocol is composed of zero-or-more activities which correspond to simple tasks that have to be followed in order to complete an experiment. Multiple users may work on the same experiment set, but only the author of an experiment set can grand another user the access to this set. The table User_experimentset_access is used for this access control purpose. Possible values of User_access_type include: a (author), r (read), and w (read-write).

Plates and Wells. An HTS experiment starts with the design of the layout of a culture Plate of $N \times M$ Wells in which the cells are kept and cultured. An experiment set can contain multiple culture plates, which typically have sizes of (but not restricted to) 4×6, 6×8 or 8×12 wells. A user can create Conditions to be applied to the wells. Similar to the Experimentset table, restricted access to the records in the Condition table are denoted explicitly in the table User_condition_access. This table keeps track of what type of access users have and which conditions are used by them in each experiment. Thus, one condition can be used in multiple experiment sets and accessed by multiple users. However, by referring to the compound primary key (User_id, Expe_id) of User_experimentset_access, a user is restricted to only have access to a condition, if he/she has access to an experiment set using the condition. Additionally, because conditions are applied on individual wells, the table Well_condition is created to store this information.

Raw Images. A third step in the HTS workflow (the "HTS" step in Figure 1) is to process the cultured plates using automated microscopy imaging system. The response of the cells is recorded through time-lapse microscopy imaging and the resulting image sequences are the basis for the image analysis. The structure of an image file depends on the type of experiment (denoted by Type_id in Experimentset) and the microscopy used in the experiment. Currently, four types of structures are supported:

1. 2D (XY): this structure corresponds to one frame containing one image which is composed of multiple channels ([1]Frame $\rightarrow$ [1]Image $\rightarrow$ [1..n]Channels).
2. 2D+T (XY+T): this structure corresponds to one video with multiple frames. Each frame contains one image composed of multiple channels ([1]Video $\rightarrow$ [1..n]Frame $\rightarrow$ [1]Image $\rightarrow$ [1..n]Channels).
3. 3D (XYZ): this structure corresponds to one frame with multiple sections. Each section contains one image composed of multiple channels ([1]Frame $\rightarrow$ [1..n] Sections $\rightarrow$ [1]Image $\rightarrow$ [1..n]Channels).
4. 3D+T (XYZ+T): this structure corresponds to one video with multiple frames. Each frame can have multiple sections and each section contains one image composed of multiple channels ([1]Video $\rightarrow$ [1..n]Frame $\rightarrow$ [1..n]Sections $\rightarrow$ [1]Image $\rightarrow$ [1..n]Channels).

These four structures can be represented by the most general one, i.e., 3D+T. The 2D structure can be seen as a video of one frame containing one section. Each frame in the 2D+T structure can regarded to contain one section. Finally, the 3D structure can be seen as a video of one frame. In the database schema, the generalised structures are captured by five relations, i.e., `Video`, `Frame`, `Section`, `Image` and `Channel`, connected to each other using foreign keys. Information stored in these relations is similar, namely a name and a description. Only the main table `Video` contains some extra information, e.g., a foreign key referring to the table `Well` to denote from which well the image has been acquired. Because currently only the metadata of the raw images are stored in these tables, the location of the image binary data is stored in `Vide_url`. The exact type of the video structure can be looked up using `Type_id` in the `Experimentset`.

Results of Image Analysis. The results of image analysis are auxiliary images which, currently, are binary masks or trajectories. These images are result of the execution of quality enhancing filters and segmentation algorithms employed to extract region of interests (ROIs). The metadata of these images is stored in the table `Measurement`, including the location where the binary data is stored. Moreover, this table also store the phenotypic measurements gathered from ROIs and trajectories, currently, as BLOBs. The foreign key `Vide_id` links a measurement record to the raw video image file, on which the image analysis has been applied.

Results of Data Analysis. Measurements extracted from the image analysis are further analysed using pattern recognition tools. Basic operations such as feature selection, clustering and classification are employed to verify the initial hypothesis or detect potential targets. The parameters used by the operation and the extracted features are respectively stored in `Parameter` and `Feature`, and are connected to the corresponding `Measurement` record via foreign keys.

5 Related Work

Data management in microscopy and cytometry has been acknowledged as an important issue. Systems have been developed to manage these resources, to this respect the Open Microscopy Environment (www.openmicroscopy.org) and the OMERO platform is a good example. Another approach is connecting all kinds of imaging data and creating a kind of virtual microscope; such has been elaborated in the Cyttron project [7] (www.cyttron.org). The connection is realized by the use of ontologies. Both projects strive at adding value to the data and allow to process the data with plug-in like packages. These approaches are very suitable for the usage of web services. Both projects are also very generic in their architecture and not particularly fit for HTS and the volume of data that is produced. Important for data management in cytometry is that both metadata and bulk data are accommodated well. The accumulation of metadata is crucial; successful accommodation of both metadata and bulk data has been applied in the field of microarrays [12]. Here, the interplay of the vendor of scanning equipment with the world of researchers in the life-sciences has delivered a standard that is proving its use in research. One cannot, one to one, copy the data model that has been applied in the field of microarrays. Like in cytometry, for microarrays the starting point is images in multiple channels. However, for cytometry, location and time components are features that are derived from the images whereas in microarrays the images are static from a template that is provided by the manufacturer. In cytometry there is a large volume of data that needs to be processed but this volume is determined by the experiment and it can be different each time; i.e. it depends very much from the experimental setup. This requires a very flexible approach to the model of the data. An important requirement for the metadata is that they can be used to link to other datasets. The use of curated concepts for annotation is part of the MAGE concept and is also embedded in the CytomicsDB project. We have successfully applied such approach for the zebrafish in which the precise annotations in the metadata were used to link out to other databases [1] and similarly, as mentioned, in the Cyttron projects the annotations are used to make direct connections within the data [7]. For cytometry data linking to other data is important in terms of interoperability so that other datasets, i.e. images, can be directly involved in an analysis. For cytometry, there are processing environments that are very much geared towards the volume of data that is commonly processed in HTS. The Konstanz Information Miner (KNIME) is a good example of such environment. It offers good functionality to process the data but it does not directly map to the workflow that is common in HTS and it does not support elaborate image analysis. Therefore, in order to be flexible, the workflow is directed towards standard packages for data processing and the processes are separated in different services rather than one service dealing with all processing. So, one service specifically for the image processing and analysis (e.g. ImageJ or DIPLIB) and another service for the pattern recognition and machine learning (e.g. WEKA or PRTools). In this manner flexibility is accomplished on the services that one can use.

6   Conclusion

In this paper we presented the design of a platform for high content data analysis in the High-Throughput Screen cytomic experiments that seamlessly connects with the workflow of the biologists and for which all processed are automated. Based on the beta testing, this system increases the efficiency of post-experiment analysis by 400%. That is, by using this the framework, it now takes less than a week to accomplish the data analysis that previously easily took more than a month with commercial software, or a year by manual observation. Comparing with solutions such as CellProfiler [5] or ImagePro, our solution provides an unique and dedicated approach for HTS image analysis. It allows end-users to perform high-profile cytomics with a minimum level of a prior experience on image analysis and machine learning. The system is modular and all modules are implemented in the form of web services, therefore, updating the system is virtually instantaneous. Moreover, the framework is very flexible as it allows connecting other web services. Consequently, a fast response to new progress in image and data analysis algorithms can be realized. Further integration with online bio-ontology databases and open gene-banks is considered so as to allow integration of the data with other resources. Therefore, the platform can eventually evolve into a sophisticated interdisciplinary platform for cytomics. Having the screen information comprehensively organized in a sophisticated and scalable database is a fertile ground for knowledge discovery.

Acknowledgements. This works is partially supported by BioRange (KY), the Erasmus BAPE program (EL), NTC (ZD) and the EU-FP7-ICT project PlanetData (http://www.planet-data.eu/).

References

1. Belmamoune, M., Verbeek, F.J.: Data integration for spatio-temporal patterns of gene expression of zebrafish development: the gems database. Journal of Integrative BioInformatics 5(2), 92 (2008)
2. Boncz, P.A.: Monet: A Next-Generation DBMS Kernel For Query-Intensive Applications. Ph.d. thesis, Universiteit van Amsterdam, Amsterdam, The Netherlands (May 2002)
3. Boncz, P.A., Manegold, S., Kersten, M.L.: Database architecture evolution: Mammals flourished long before dinosaurs became extinct. PVLDB 2(2), 1648–1653 (2009)
4. Cao, L., Yan, K., Winkel, L., de Graauw, M., Verbeek, F.J.: Pattern Recognition in High-Content Cytomics Screens for Target Discovery - Case Studies in Endocytosis. In: Loog, M., Wessels, L., Reinders, M.J.T., de Ridder, D. (eds.) PRIB 2011. LNCS, vol. 7036, pp. 330–342. Springer, Heidelberg (2011)
5. Carpenter, A., Jones, T., Lamprecht, M., Clarke, C., Kang, I., Friman, O., Gertin, D., Chang, J., Lindquist, R., Moffat, J., Golland, P., Sabatini, D.: Cellprofiler: image analysis software for identifying and quantifying cell phenotypes. Genome Biology 7(10) (2006)
6. Gudgin, M., Mendelsohn, N., Nottingham, M., Ruellan, H.: Soap message transmission optimization mechanism (2005)
7. Kallergi, A., Bei, Y., Kok, P., Dijkstra, J., Abrahams, J., Verbeek, F.: Cyttron: A virtualized microscope supporting image integration and knowledge discovery. Cell Death and Disease Series: Proteins Killing Tumour Cells, pp. 291–315 (2009)
8. LeDévédec, S., Yan, K., de Bont, H., Ghotra, V., Truong, H., Danen, E., Verbeek, F., van de Water, B.: A systems microscopy approach to understand cancer cell migration and metastasis. Journal of Cellular and Molecular in Life Science (2010)
9. MATLAB. version 7.10.0 (R2010a). The MathWorks Inc., Natick, Massachusetts (2010)
10. Neumann, B., Walter, T., Hériché, J., Bulkescher, J., Erfle, H., Conrad, C., Rogers, P., Poser, I., Held, M., Liebel, U., Cetin, C., Sieckmann, F., Pau, G., Kabbe, R., Wünsche, A., Satagopam, V., Schmitz, M., Chapuis, C., Gerlich, D., Schneider, R., Eils, R., Huber, W., Peters, J., Hyman, A., Durbin, R., Pepperkok, R., Ellenberg, J.: Phenotypic profiling of the human genome by time-lapse microscopy reveals cell division genes. Nature 464(7289), 721–727 (2010)
11. Qin, Y., Stokman, G., Yan, K., Ramaiahgari, S., Verbeek, F., van de Water, B., Price, L.: Activation of epac-rap signaling protects against cisplatin-induced apoptosis of mouse renal proximal tubular cells. Journal of Biological Chemistry (2011) (in Press)
12. Spellman, P., Miller, M., Stewart, J., Troup, C., Sarkans, U., Chervitz, S., Bernhart, D., Sherlock, G., Ball, C., Lepage, M., Swiatek, M., Marks, W., Goncalves, J., Markel, S., Iordan, D., Shojatalab, M., Pizarro, A., White, J., Hubley, R., Deutsch, E., Senger, M., Aronow, B., Robinson, A., Bassett, D., Stoeckert, C., Brazma, A.: Design and implementation of microarray gene expression markup language (mage-ml). Genome Biology 3(9), RESEARCH0046 (2002)
13. Yan, K., Larios, E., LeDévédec, S., van de Water, B., Verbeek, F.: Automation in cytomics: Systematic solution for image analysis and management in high throughput sequences. In: Proceedings IEEE Conf. Engineering and Technology (CET 2011), vol. 7, pp. 195–198 (2011)
14. Yan, K., LeDévédec, S., van de Water, B., Verbeek, F.: Cell tracking and data analisys of in vitro tumour cells from time-lapse image sequences. In: VISAPP 2009 (2009)

MRF Reconstruction of Retinal Images for the Optic Disc Segmentation

Ana Salazar-Gonzalez*, Yongmin Li, and Djibril Kaba

Brunel Universit, Department of Information Systems and Computer Science,
UB8 3PH Uxbridge, London
http://www.brunel.ac.uk/

Abstract. The retinal image analysis has been of great interest because of its efficiency and reliability for optical diagnosis. Different techniques have been designed for the segmentation of the eye structures and lesions. In this paper we present an unsupervised method for the segmentation of the optic disc. Blood vessels represent the main obstruction in the optic disc segmentation process. We made use of our previous work in blood vessel segmentation to perform an image reconstruction using the Markov Random Field formulation (MRF). As a result the optic disc appears as a well defined structure. A traditional graph is then constructed using spatial pixel connections as boundary term and the likelihood of the pixels belonging to the foreground and background seeds as regional term. Our algorithm was implemented and tested on two public data sets, DIARETDB1 and DRIVE. The results are evaluated and compared with other methods in the literature.

Keywords: Retinal image, segmentation, optic disc, retinal lesions.

1 Introduction

The segmentation of medical images constitutes the first step for different analyses such as anatomical structures, tissues and computer assisted diagnosis. Due to poor contrast, weak boundary definition and inconsistent elements, medical images are challenging to analyse and require further studies.

The optic disc can be described as the brightest round area where the blood vessels converge. This convergence feature is often used to localize the optic disc. At the same time blood vessels constitute the first obstruction for the optic disc segmentation breaking the continuity of the object to segment. Some techniques have addressed the vessels intrusion using morphological operations as preprocessing [5, 11].

In this paper we present an unsupervised method for the segmentation of the optic disc. The main contribution of this paper is the use of prior segmented vessel to perform the reconstruction of the retinal image, as a result the optic

* The authors would like to thank the Mexican National Council for Science and Technology (CONACYT) for financial support, and to Yun Zeng for his contribution to produce the segmentation results using the topology cut technique.

J. He et al. (Eds.): HIS 2012, LNCS 7231, pp. 88–99, 2012.

disc appears as a well defined structure. Assuming the blood vessel pixels as unknown, the retinal image is reconstructed using MRF formulation. The reconstructed image presents better edge definition of the optic disc improving the segmentation results. Later the Graph Cut technique is used to segment the optic disc on the reconstructed image. The graph is initialized automatically using the MRF reconstructed image.

The rest of the paper is organised as follows. Section 2 makes a review of the current methods for the location and segmentation of the optic disc in the literature. Section 3 is dedicated to describe our method. We have included details about the MRF reconstruction performed on the retinal image by using prior segmented vessels. Finally experimental results are presented in section 4.

2   Background

In [3] a combination of morphological operations, Hough transform and an anchored active contour model is used to segment the optic disc. The blood vessels are removed by using a distance map; each pixel is assigned a value equal to its distance from the nearest boundary. This distance map is then thresholded and all pixels with a distance of six or less are removed. The method assumes a maximum vessel diameter of ten pixels, which produce a distance of five, but this is not always the case for all retinal images datasets. A deformable contour model is used to segment the optic disc in [7]. The model makes use of a direction-sensitive gradient which try to ignore vessel edges distraction. The watershed transform form markers is used to find the optic disc boundary in [11]. A first boundary is found by using initial makers, later by using an iterative process markers are updated and new boundary is defined. In order to minimize the vessel obstruction in the internal marker the method performs morphological erosion. In [5] the optic disc boundary is localized by using morphological and edges detection techniques followed by a Circular Hough Transform. The authors consider the blood vessels within the optic disc as a strong distracter and indicate that they should be erased. The method makes use of morphological processing to eliminate vessels.

In [12] blood vessels are used to estimate the location of the optic disc. The retinal vessels are segmented by using a 2-D Gaussian matched filter and a vessel direction map is created. The vessels are then thinned, and filtered using local intensity, to finally represent the optic disc centre candidates. The minimum difference between the matched filter result and the vessel direction around each candidate provides an estimation of the optic disc location. The method just localize the optic disc, but it does not perform its segmentation.

In [9] the histogram of the enhanced retinal image is modelled using a mixture model. From the histogram shape, two heavy tails are distinguished and assumed as foreground area (vessels, optic disc and lesions). It is assumed that the high intensity tail includes the optic disc. From the high intensity tail optic disc is segmented. The segmentation is performed by using mathematical morphology to select candidate pixels; this selection is then prune by restricting the selection to the pixels in the neighbourhood of the main vessels. The main vessels are detected by using a two dimensional vertical oriented filter. The method assumes that the primary four vessels normally emanate near vertically from the optic disc. This assumption limited the performance of this method to the type of retinal images where the optic disc has been captured under the exact conditions to clearly display the four main vessels crossing vertically the optic disc.

Morphological operations are a recursive element to eliminate vessels from the retinal image beforehand [11, 5]. But this type of processing operates not only on vessels, the modification is extended to the rest of the image and some important information can be corrupted. This issue has been pointed out in [5], which declares that as a consequence of this processing the optic disc is enlarged by a fixed length in all directions.

In our discrimination of vessels method we remove vessels from the ROI by using prior vessel segmentation to perform the reconstruction of the image. The reconstruction is performed only on the vessel pixels (unknown pixels) to avoid the modification of other structures. Our proposed methods were designed as unsupervised methods, and they can perform on images with different characteristics. In the next section the process to localize the optic disc is explained. Next, the problem of segmenting overlapping tissues is presented and the methods to explore the opposing research lines are detailed.

3 Our Method

The retinal blood vessels have two roles in the optic disc segmentation. On one hand they are the main obstruction when segmenting the optic disc; and on the other hand blood vessels inside the optic disc are part of the object to segment. We start a MRF reconstruction of the retinal image from a previous blood vessel segmentation. Blood vessel pixels are considered as unknown and the surrounded pixels are used to fill these vacancies. We have selected a Markov Random Field based reconstruction technique. The general idea is to find the best matching for the missing pixels. One of the disadvantages of this approach is the intensive time consumption. We address this problem by limiting the reconstruction to a smaller area of the image that contains the region of interest. The method is described in Table 1.

Table 1. The optic disc segmentation

Input: Colour retinal image I_{in}
1. Segment the blood vessels from I_{in} [8];
2. I_c = Localize the optic disc and constrain the image;
3. I_r = Perform the MRF reconstruction of I_c;
4. Initialize Fg_s and Bg_s in I_r;
5. I_{out} = Construct graph for I_r and resolve;
Output: Optic disc segmented I_{out}

In the first stage blood vessels are segmented from the retinal colour image. The blood vessels convergence is localized and assumed as the center of the optic disc. The retinal image is then constrained to the region of interest and the MRF reconstruction is performed using the prior blood vessel segmentation. Foreground Fg_s and background Bg_s seeds are initialized in the reconstructed image and used to construct the graph. Finally the graph is cut by minimizing the energy function and producing the optimal segmentation of the image.

3.1   Blood Vessels Segmentation

As a first step eye structures are segmented. We have selected the graph cut technique for this purpose. Graph cut is an interactive image segmentation technique in computer vision and medical image analysis [1]. Graph cut methods have been used widely in image segmentation due to its ability to compute globally optimal solutions. The general idea is to map an image onto a graph with weighted connections. The graph is then cut (separating foreground and background), minimizing the energy function and producing the optimal segmentation for the image.

The graph cut based method [8] is adopted in this work. First the green channel of the retinal colour image is enhanced. An improved adaptive histogram equalization is applied to the image, followed by a pruning stage in order to obtain a rough segmentation of the vessels. The distant transform is calculated from the binary resultant image. The flux of the vectors in the distant map along with regional boundaries terms are used to construct a graph. Finally the graph is cut, resulting in the segmentation of the blood vessels.

3.2   Optic Disc Location

Once the vessel network is segmented, the image is pruned using a morphologic open operation in order to keep the main arcade of the vessels. Inspired by the work presented in [11] the centroid of the arcade is calculated using:

$$C_x = \sum_{i=1}^{K} \frac{x_i}{K} \qquad C_y = \sum_{i=1}^{K} \frac{y_i}{K} \qquad (1)$$

where x_i and y_i are the coordinates of the pixel in the binary image and K is the number of pixels set to "1", which is the pixels marked as blood vessels in the binary image.

Using the blue channel of the RGB retinal image, the 1% of the brigthest pixels are marked. The algorithm detects the brightest area in the image in order to determine the position of the optic disc with respect to the centroid. This is followed by a pruning to eliminate the group of pixels with fewer elements. In order to find the most likely center of the optic disc our algorithm finds the way from the centroid to the vessels convergence by adjusting the point while approaching. Considering that the main arcade is narrowing until the vessels converge, the algorithm adjusts the centroid point by reducing the distance with the optic disc and keeping the same distance with the vessel on the main arcade. Figure 1 shows an example of optic disc detection.

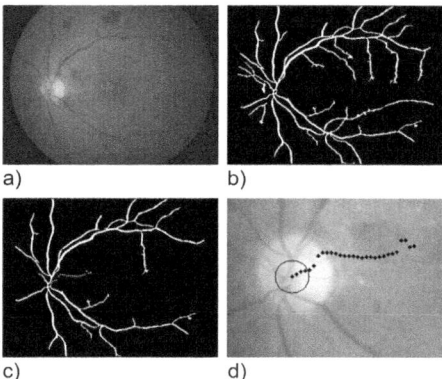

Fig. 1. Optic disc detection. a) retinal image, b) blood vessel segmentation, c) blood vessel segmentation after pruning and d) sequence of points from the centroid to the vessels convergence.

Our algorithm detected successfully 96.7% of the DIARETDB1 [6] data set images and in 97.5% of the images in DRIVE [10]. We constrain the image to a smaller area in order to minimize processing time. The region of interest is constrained to a square of 200 by 200 pixels concentric with the optic disc.

3.3   Optic Disc Segmentation

In order to produce an image with a well defined optic disc, the retinal image is reconstructed using a prior blood vessel segmentation. We have selected a Markov Random Field based method to perform the reconstruction [4]. Blood vessel pixels are considered as unknown. The general idea is to find a collection of patches statistically similar to the patch where a pixel p $(p = 0)$ is missed. Then we create a histogram of the pixels that are in the same position as p in the collection of patches and obtain the best approximate value to substitute the missing pixel.

A pixel neighborhood $w(p)$ is defined as a square window of size W, with center on pixel p. The image that is going to be reconstructed is I. Some of the pixels in I are missing and the objective is to find the best approximate value for them. Let $d(w1, w2)$ indicate a perceptual distance between two patches that indicate how likely they are. The exact matching patch would be the one that $d(w', w(p)) = 0$. If we define a set of these patches as $\Omega(p) = \{\omega' \subset I : d(\omega', \omega(p)) = 0\}$ the probability density function of p can be estimated with a histogram of all center pixel values in $\Omega(p)$. But owing to the fact that we are considering a finite neighborhood for p and the searching is limited to the image area, there might not be any exact matches for the patch. For this reason in our implementation we find a collection of patches whose match falls between the best match and a threshold. The closest match is calculated as $\omega_{best} = argmin_\omega d(\omega(p), \omega) \subset I$. And all the patches ω with $d(\omega(p), \omega) < (1 + \epsilon)d(\omega(p), \omega_{best})$ are included in the collection ω'. In our implementation $d(w', w(p))$ is defined as the sum of the absolute differences of the intensities between patches, so identical patches will result in $d(w', w(p)) = 0$. We have set $\epsilon = 0.1$ and $W = 5$. Using the collection of patches we create a histogram and select the one with highest mode. The reconstruction process is summarized in Table 2 and Figure 2 shows some examples of reconstructed images.

Table 2. Pseudo function for the MRF image reconstruction in the constrained retinal image

Inputs: Retinal gray scale image I_g and binary blood vessel image I_{bv}.
1. If $I_{bv}(p) = vessel$ then $I_g(p) = 0$;   2. Create a list of unknown pixels p in I_g, 　　$I_g(p) = 0$ and their neighborhood $w(p)$;   3. Sort out the list according with the number of 　　unknown pixels included as part of the neighborhood $w(p)$;   4. for $i = 0$ to $i = W - 1$; 　　for each element in the list; 　　patch $= $ w(p) if unknown neighbors number is equal to i; 　　find $\omega_{best} = argmin_\omega d(\omega(p), \omega) \subset I$; 　　collection of patches $d(\omega(p), \omega) < (1 + \epsilon)d(\omega(p), \omega_{best})$; 　　create a histogram of collection of patches; 　　Substitute p in I_g by the intensity with highest mode; 　　$i + +$ 　　end for 　end for

Foreground and Background Seeds Initialization. Using the retinal reconstructed image, the foreground Fg_s and background Bg_s seeds are initialized. A neighborhood of 20 pixels of radius around the centre of the optic disc is marked as Fg_s pixels, while a band of pixels around the perimeter of the image are taken as Bg_s.

Graph for Optic Disc Segmentation. Graph cut is a well known technique used for interactive image segmentation in computer vision and more specific in medical image analysis [2, 14]. The general idea is to map the image into a graph with weighted connections. The graph is then cut (separating foreground and background) by minimizing the energy function and producing the optimal segmentation for the image. For the optic disc segmentation we have selected the traditional edge weight assignment method as presented in [1]. The energy function consists of regional and boundary terms. Regional term is calculated

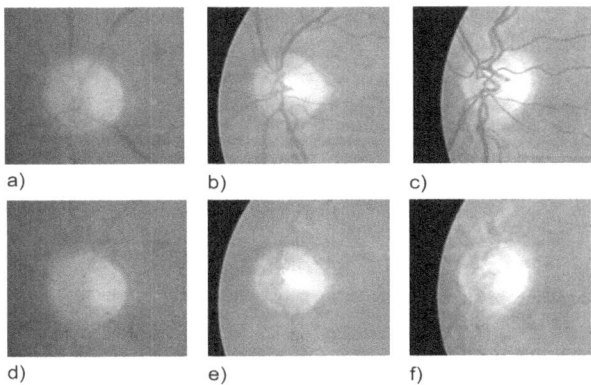

Fig. 2. MRF reconstruction applied to retinal images. (Top) original gray scale images. (Bottom) reconstructed images using the MRF based method.

from the likelihood of a pixel p belonging to the foreground and background, generating the t-links weight. The boundary term is based on the own pixel properties (i.e. intensity) which is used to assign weight to the n-links.

A grid of 16 neighbors N is selected to create links between pixels in the image Im. The n-links and t-links weights are assigned according to Table 3. lik_{Fg} and lik_{Bg} represent the negative log-likelihood of the pixel p with respect to the prior information of the foreground and background. The distance $dist(p, q)$ is defined by the Euclidean distance between p and q. Max-Flow[1] is used to cut the graph and find the optimal segmentation.

Table 3. Link weight assignment for the graph of the optic disc segmentation process

link	weight	for
n-link	$B_{p,q}$	$p, q \in N$
t-link (Foreground)	$\lambda \cdot lik_{Fg}$	$p \in Im, p \notin F \cup B$
	K	$p \in F$
	0	$p \in B$
t-link (Background)	$\lambda \cdot lik_{Bg}$	$p \in Im, p \notin F \cup B$
	0	$p \in F$
	K	$p \in B$

$$\text{where } B_{p,q} = exp(-\frac{(I_p - I_q)^2}{2\sigma^2}) \cdot \frac{1}{dist(p,q)}$$
$$K = 1 + max_{p \in Im} \sum_q B_{p,q}$$

4   Results

Our method was tested on two public data sets, DIARETDB1 (89 images) [6] and DRIVE (40 images) [10]. We created hand labeled sets for DIARETDB1 and

---

[1] maxflow-v3.01 is available at
http://www.cs.ucl.ac.uk/staff/V.Kolmogorov/software.html.

DRIVE in order to have a ground truth to compare our results. The performance of the methods was evaluated by the overlapping ratio (*Oratio*) and the mean absolute distance(*MAD*). The overlapping ratio is defined as:

$$Oratio = \frac{G \bigcap S}{G \bigcup S}$$

where G represents the manually segmented area and S is the area as result of the algorithm segmentation. MAD is defined as:

$$MAD(G_c, S_c) = \frac{1}{2} \left\{ \frac{1}{n} \sum_{i=1}^{n} d(g_{c_i}, S) + \frac{1}{m} \sum_{i=1}^{m} d(s_{c_i}, G) \right\}$$

where G_c and S_c are the contour of the segmented area in the ground truth and the resulting images, and $d(a_i, B)$ is the minimum distance from the position of the pixel a_i on the contour A to the contour B. A good segmentation implies a high overlapping ratio and a low MAD value.

We calculated the sensitivity of the methods when they are applied to DI-ARETDB1 and DRIVE, which is defined as:

$$Sensitivity = \frac{Tp}{Tp + Fn}$$

where Tp and Fn are the number of true positives and the number of false negatives respectively. Sensitivity is an indicator of the foreground pixels detected by the segmentation method.

Our results are compared to those provided in [11]. This method was tested on the same datasets (DIARETDB1 and DRIVE) and results were measured under the same parameters. Also we have included the results of our experiments using the traditional graph cut technique without compensation and the ones using the topology cut technique [13].

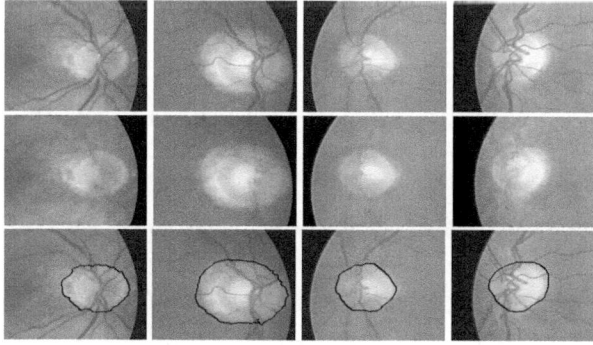

Fig. 3. Optic disc segmentation results. First row: original image, second row: MRF reconstructed image, third row: optic disc segmentation.

Unfortunately most of the methods do not use a unique ground truth to measure the results of the optic disc segmentation, so this makes the comparison of the results difficult.

Figure 3 shows the segmentation results on images with and without reconstruction. We have included sample images of both data sets with different *Oratio* measures. It is clear that a significant improvement has been achieved when the images have been reconstructed previously using the MRF formulation.

Figures 4, 5 and 6 show the segmentation results on the DIARETDB1 and DRIVE datasets by using three different methods, traditional graph cut technique, topology cut technique and our method. The segmentation results are evaluated in terms of the *Oratio* by using the ground truth images. The graph cut segmentation improves considerably when it is applied to a well defined optic disc. When the MRF reconstruction was applied the segmentation improved in 95% of the images on DRIVE, and 80% of the images on DIARETDB1.

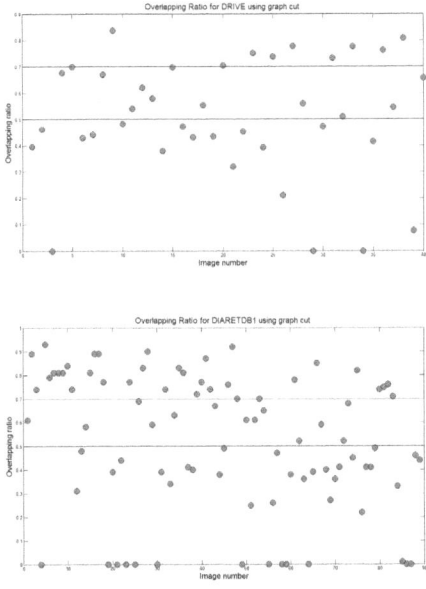

Fig. 4. Optic disc segmentation results on the DIARETDB1 and DRIVE datasets by using Graph Cut technique

There are few specific cases where the segmentation of the optic disc resulted in null. This cases are shared by the other methods as well. The characteristic of these images is the poor contrast, as a consequence all the pixels are linked with strong weight and is not possible to find a cut to segment it. This is an indication of the challenge of analyzing those specific images.

Table 4 and Table 5 show the comparison with different methods in terms of *Oratio*, *MAD* and *Sensitivity*. Our method achieved the highest overlapping

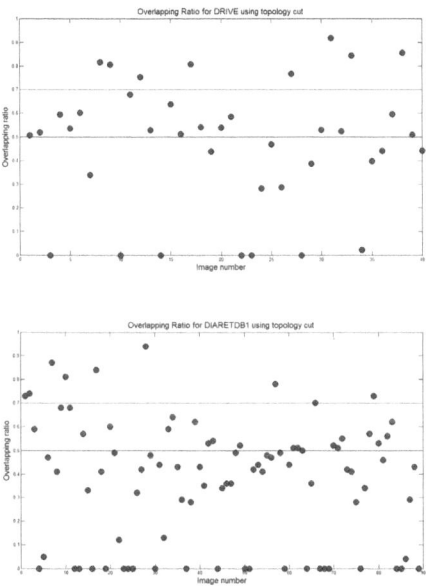

Fig. 5. Optic disc segmentation results on the DIARETDB1 and DRIVE datasets by using Topology Cut technique

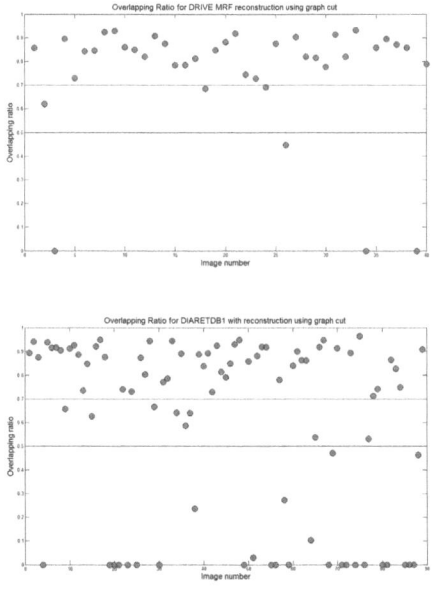

Fig. 6. Optic disc segmentation results on the DIARETDB1 and DRIVE datasets by using our method

ratio with the minimum MAD value. It can be seen that an increase in the overlapping ratio does not mean a decrease on MAD value necessarily. MAD value does not represent the best way to measure the segmentation results, but it provides a good reference of the contour matching with the ground truth contour reference.

Table 4. Performance comparison on the DIARETDB1 dataset

Method	Average ORatio	Average MAD	Average Sensitivity
Topoly Cut	38.43%	17.49	55.30%
Adaptive morphologic [11]	43.65%	8.31	—
Graph Cut	54.03%	10.74	76.35%
MRF + Graph Cut	78.3%	6.75	87.3%

Table 5. Performance comparison on the DRIVE dataset

Method	Average ORatio	Average MAD	Average Sensitivity
Topoly Cut	55.91%	10.24	65.12%
Adaptive morphologic [11]	41.47%	5.74	—
Graph Cut	55.32%	9.97	73.98%
MRF + Graph Cut	82.2%	3.59	97.99%

It is possible appreciate that our method performs better on the DRIVE dataset. The 95.5% of the images in DIARETDB1 dataset are characterized by contain at least one type of retinal lesion. In general, a healthy retinal image is easier to analyse than a image with some type of retinopathy.

5   Conclusions

Optic disc segmentation is an important process in the analysis of retinal images. The analysis of optic disc morphology is part of the retinal screen process. Retinal Blood vessel network requires special attention due to its overlapping with the optic disc.

In this paper we have presented an unsupervised method for the segmentation of the optic disc. Our method performs MRF reconstruction by using prior segmented vessels. Vessels are masked out and a well defined optic disc is created.

Our method was tested on two public data sets: DIARETDB1 and DRIVE. Experimental results were compared with other methods, including the traditional formulation of the graph cut and the topology cut techniques. The results comparison shows the outperformance of our method.

References

1. Boykov, Y., Funka-Lea, G.: Graph cuts and efficient n-d image segmentation. International Journal of Computer Vision 70(2), 109–131 (2006)
2. Chittajallu, D.R., Brunner, G., Kurkure, U., Yalamanchili, R.P., Kakadiaris, I.A.: Fuzzy-cuts: A knowledge-driven graph-based method for medical image segmentation. In: Proceedings of the Twenty Third IEEE Coference on Computer, Vision and Pattern Recognition, pp. 715–722 (2009)
3. Chrastek, R., Wolf, M., Donath, K., Niemann, H., Paulus, D., Hothorn, T., Lausen, B., Lammer, R., Mardin, C.Y., Michelson, G.: Automated segmentation of the optic nerve head for diagnosis of glaucoma. Medical Image Analysis 9(1), 297–314 (2005)
4. Efros, A.A., Leung, T.K.: Texture synthesis by non-parametric sampling. In: Proceedings of the ICCV, pp. 1033–1038 (1999)
5. Aquino, A., et al.: Detecting the optic disc boundary in digital fundus images using morphological, edge detection and feature extraction techniques. IEEE Transactions on Medical Imaging 29(10), 1860–1869 (2010)
6. Kauppi, T., Kalesnykiene, V., Kamarainen, J., Lensu, L., Sorri, I., Raninen, A., Voitilainen, R., Uusitalo, H., Kalviainen, H., Pietila, J.: Diaretdb1 diabetic retinopathy database and evaluation protocol. In: Proceedings of British Machine Vision Conference (2007)
7. Lowell, J., Hunter, A., Steel, D., Basu, A., Ryder, R., Fletcher, E., Kennedy, L.: Optic nerve head segmentation. IEEE Transactions on Medical Imaging 23(2), 256–264 (2004)
8. Salazar-Gonzalez, A., Li, Y., Liu, X.: Retinal blood vessel segmentation via graph cut. In: Proceedings of the 11th International Conference on Control, Automation, Robotics and Vision, ICARCV, vol. 1, pp. 225–230 (2010)
9. Sanchez, C.I., Garcia, M., Mayo, A., Lopez, M.I., Hornero, R.: Retinal image analysis based on mixture models to detect hard exudates. Medical Image Analysis 13, 650–658 (2009)
10. Staal, J., Abramoff, M.D., Niemeijer, M., Viergever, M.A., van Ginneken, B.: Ridge-based vessel segmentation in color images of the retina. IEEE Transactions on Medical Imaging 23(4), 501–509 (2004)
11. Welfer, D., Scharcanski, J., Kitamura, C., Dal Pizzol, M., Ludwig, L., Marinho, D.: Segmentation of the optic disc in color eye fundus images using an adaptive morphological approach. Computers in Biology and Medicine 40(1), 124–137 (2010)
12. Youssif, A., Ghalwash, A., Ghoneim, A.: Optic disc detection from normalized digital fundus images by means of a vessels's directed matched filter. IEEE Transactions on Medical Imaging 27(1), 11–18 (2008)
13. Zeng, Y., Samaras, D., Chen, W., Peng, Q.: Topology cuts: a novel min-cut/max-flow algorithm for topology preserving segmentation in n-d images. Journal of computer vision and image understanding 112(1), 81–90 (2008)
14. Zhu-Jacquot, J., Zabih, R.: Graph cuts segmentation with statistical shape prior for medical image. In: Proceedings of the Third International IEEE Conference on Signal-Image Technologies and Internet-Based System, pp. 631–635 (2008)

Normalized Cut Segmentation of Thyroid Tumor Image Based on Fractional Derivatives

Jie Zhao[1], Li Zhang[1], Wei Zheng[1], Hua Tian[1], Dong-mei Hao[2], and Song-hong Wu[2]

[1] College of Electronic and Information Engineering of Hebei University,
Baoding, 071002, China
Zhaojie_hbu@126.com
[2] Affiliated hospital of Hebei University, Baoding, 071002, China

Abstract. In the clinical diagnosis of thyroid tumor, ultrasound image may provide anatomical detail of the tumor, and radionuclide image may provide functional information about activity distribution of the tumor. Fusion of the two-modality medical image doesn't only supply more abundant and comprehensive pathology information for clinic diagnosis, but also reduce the radioactive hazard from ionizing radiation because of multiple scans of x-rays of Computed Tomography. In order to realize the registration and fusion of the two modality images, we must segment the thyroid and surrounding tissues. Most of original medical images are poor contrast and intensity inhomogeneous. Hence, it is very difficult to segment using traditional segmental methods. A novel normalized cut segmentation method based on fractional derivatives is proposed and applied into thyroid tumor images in this paper. In our proposed method, the thought of fractional derivatives is introduced to implement normalized cut, which enhances thyroid tumor images by adjusting the fractional derivatives parameters, marking edge and raising the accuracy. The results of experiments show feasibility and effectiveness of proposed method.

Keywords: Fractional derivatives, normalized cut, thyroid tumor image, image segmentation.

1 Introduction

The thyroid gland is one of the largest endocrine glands. The thyroid gland is found in the neck, below the thyroid cartilage. The isthmus of the thyroid (the bridge between the two lobes of the thyroid) is located inferior to the cricoid cartilage. The thyroid gland controls how quickly the body uses energy, produces proteins, and controls how sensitive the body is to other hormones. It participates in these processes by producing thyroid hormones, such as triiodothyronine (T3) and thyroxine (T4). Thyroid cancer is a malignant tumor that develops in the tissue of the thyroid gland, which destroys function of thyroid and threats to life of patient. The most common presenting symptom is a painless mass. It is very unusual for the thyroid cancers to present with particular symptoms, unless it has been diagnosed. One may feel a hard

J. He et al. (Eds.): HIS 2012, LNCS 7231, pp. 100–109, 2012.

nodule in the neck. Diagnosis is made using a needle biopsy and various radiological studies [1].

Needle aspiration biopsy (NAB), also known as fine needle aspiration cytology (FNAC), fine needle aspiration biopsy (FNAB) and fine needle aspiration (FNA), is a diagnostic procedure sometimes used to investigate superficial lumps or masses. In this technique, a thin and hollow needle is inserted into the mass to sample cells which will be examined under a microscope after being stained. There could be cytology exam of aspirate (cell specimen evaluation, FNAC) or histological (biopsy - tissue specimen evaluation, FNAB). A needle aspiration biopsy is safer and less traumatic than open surgical biopsy. The significant complications are usually rare, strong related with physique of patients. Common complications include bruising and soreness. There mainly exist two risks: (1)Because the biopsy is very small (only a few cells), the problematic cells may be missed, and false negative result may be gotten. (2)The cells taken will not enable a definitive diagnosis[2].

Various radiological technologies used to study thyroid tumor include projectional radiographs(x-rays), magnetic resonance imaging (MRI) , Computed Tomography (CT), Single-photon emission computed tomography (SPECT, or less commonly, SPET) and Positron emission tomography(PET). Projection radiographs are often used to determine the type and extent of a fracture and detect pathological changes in the lungs. This imaging modality utilizes a wide beam of x rays for image acquisition, involving the use of ionizing radiation. Therefore, it's not associated with the same health hazards. A magnetic resonance imaging instrument (MRI scanner) emits an RF (radio frequency) pulse that specifically binds only to hydrogen. Modern MRI instruments are capable of producing images in the form of 3D blocks. However, there are well-identified health risks associated with tissue heating from exposure to the RF field. Computed Tomography (CT) uses X-rays and has a greater ionizing radiation dose burden than projection radiography. Scan number must be limited to avoid health effects. CT is based on the same principles as X-Ray projections but patients are enclosed in a surrounding ring of detectors assigned with 500-1000 scintillation detectors (fourth-generation X-Ray CT scanner geometry). Previously in older generation scanners, the X-Ray beam was paired by a translating source and detector. Medical ultrasonography uses high frequency broadband sound waves in the megahertz range that are reflected by tissue to varying degrees to produce (up to 3D) images. While it may provide less anatomical detail than techniques such as CT or MRI, it has several advantages which make it ideal in numerous situations, in particular that it studies the function of moving structures in real-time, emits no ionizing radiation, and contains speckle that can be used in elastography. It is very safe to use and does not appear to cause any adverse effects, although information on this is not well documented. It is also relatively inexpensive and quick to perform. Nuclear medicine encompasses both diagnostic imaging and treatment of disease, and may also be referred to as molecular medicine or molecular imaging & therapeutics. This function-based approach to medical evaluation has useful applications in most subspecialties, notably oncology, neurology, and cardiology. Gamma cameras are used in e.g. scintigraphy, SPECT and PET to detect regions of biologic activity that may be associated with disease. Images are acquired after collimated photons are detected by a crystal that gives off a light signal, which is in turn amplified and converted into count data [3].

Various kind of advanced medical imaging equipments supply multi-modality medical images. Medical images in different modality display different characteristic information of human viscera and pathological changed tissue. Multi-modality medical image fusion is that use image fusion technology in medical images, in order to supply more abundant pathology information for clinic diagnoses [4]. Today, the fusion technologies inculde SPECT and CT, SPECT and MRI, health hazards from ionizing radiation or RF field cannot be avoided.

Therefore, it is very significant that functional information from SPECT can be related to anatomical information provided by Ultrasound to diagnose thyroid tumor. Ultrasound scanners can be applied to patients in intensive care units, avoiding risk caused while moving the patient to the radiology department. In SPECT imaging, the patient is injected with a radioisotope, most commonly Thallium 201TI, Technetium 99mTC, Iodine 123I, and Gallium 67Ga. The emissions of the gamma rays are captured by detectors that surround the body. Images of activity distribution throughout the body can show rapidly growing tissue, like tumor, metastasis, or infection [5]. In future, a SPECT/ Ultrasound camera can be designed and made .

In order to realize feature level fusion of Ultrasound images and radionuclide images from SPECT, it is critical to accurately segment the two kinds of images of thyroid tumor. Image segmentation is the technology and the process of dividing and image into some areas and extracting the interesting target. Image segmentation is widely used in computer aided diagnosis, pathological analysis, medical plan and so on. The accuracy of the segmentation determines the eventual success or failure of computerized analysis procedure [6]. According to the features of the images, a novel algorithm, normalized cut based on fractional derivatives, is proposed to segment the thyroid tumor. Experimental results show that the proposed algorithm shows better performance than traditional segmental algorithm.

2   Principle of the Algorithm

A Ultrasound image of thyroid tumor of a patient is shown in Fig.1(a), and radionuclide image of the patient is shown in Fig.1(b).

Because of the limitations in the imaging devices and subject-induced susceptibility effect, the obtained images are poor contrast and intensity inhomogeneous. Hence these problems have made it more difficult for the traditional segmentation method to segment accurately and efficiently. Traditional image segmentation approaches mainly include threshold technique, edge detecting algorithms and region-based methods. Threshold technique ignoring spatial information can create meaningless region boundaries. Edge detection is mainly used to segment images base on abrupt changes in intensity. Detecting changes for the purpose of finding edges can be accomplished using first-order or second-order derivatives. Edge detecting technique can lead to broken boundary lines and consequently must be combined with boundary tracing technique. To region-based technique, it is very difficult to design an appropriate criterion for splitting and merging in the procedure of processing low contrast images. Mathematical morphology, as the foundation of morphological image processing, is a theory and technique for the analysis and processing of geometrical structures, based on set theory, lattice theory, topology and random functions. The morphological segmentation algorithm of watershed transform has been successfully applied to many fields including medical and military. But, it often results in oversegmentation to use watershed transform directly on an original image. A graph-cut is a grouping technique in which the degree of dissimilarity between these two groups is computed as the total weight of edges removed between these 2 pieces. In grouping, a weighted graph is split into disjoint sets (groups) where by some measure the similarity within a group is high and that across the group is low. By minimizing this cut value, one can optimally bi-partition the graph and achieve good segmentation. Normalized cut computes the cut cost as a fraction of the total edge connections to all the nodes in the graph. The normalized cut criterion measures both the total dissimilarity between the different groups as well as the total similarity within the groups [7]. According to characteristics of Ultrasound image and radionuclear image, an improved Normalized Cut algorithm is proposed. It is a normalized cut algorithm based on the fractional differential. It introduces the fractional derivatives into the normalized cut, and enhances thyroid tumor images by adjusting the fractional derivatives parameters, marking the outline of images and accurately calculating the weight matrix, further segmenting the areas of thyroid tumor through the discrete eigenvectors. The result of experiment shows the feasibility of the algorithm.

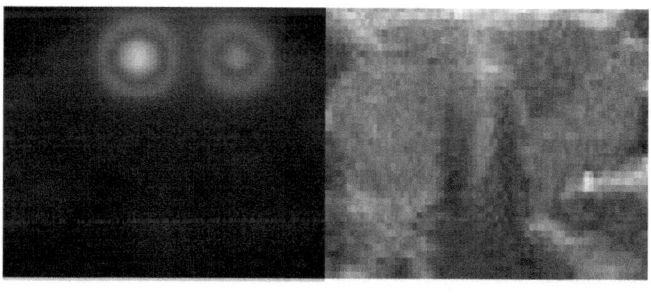

(a) ultrasonic image   (b) radionuclide image

Fig. 1. Original image of thyroid tumor

3   Image Enhancement Based on Fractional Differential

Producing spot make the image poor quality with noise in the process of formating ultrasonic images and shape characteristic of radionuclide image is irregular and its organization boundary is fuzzy. So according to the characteristics of thyroid imaging, we construct the fractional differential mask operator with four directions[8], put their maximum as fractional differential pixel gray value, and add with the original image to get the enhancing image by superposition with improved image[9]. Detecting edge of enhance images to get edge figures and getting the weight matrix according to edge figures, finally segment thyroid tumor images using the eigenvectors.

Image enhancement processes image for improving the quality of image for the application purpose and strengthen characteristics interested in the image. Based on the characteristics of fractional differential with improving high frequency component of signal[10], enhancing intermediate frequency components of signal, nonlinearly retaining the vlf-component of the signal, we introduce fractional differential into fields of image enhancement. Compared with the traditional image enhancement algorithms, it strengthens the detail information of high frequency texture for thyroid tumor image and maintains overall outline information.

The duration of one source $f(t)$ is $t \in [a,t]$, parting the duration as unit interval $h = 1$, so $n = [\frac{t-a}{h}]^{h=1} = [t-a]$, then derived difference expression of one source $f(t)$ fractional derivatives [11].

$$\frac{d^v f(t)}{dt^v} \approx f(t) + (-v)f(t-1) + \frac{(-v)(-v+1)}{2}f(t-2) + \frac{(-v)(-v+1)}{6}f(t-2)$$
$$+ \frac{(-v)(-v+1)(-v+2)}{6}f(t-3) + \cdots + \frac{\Gamma(-v+1)}{n!\Gamma(-v+n+1)}f(t-n) \tag{1}$$

Filter images with the $m*n$ size masking of filter linearly, getting from formula (2).

$$g(x,y) = \sum_{s=-a}^{a} \sum_{t=-b}^{b} w(s,t)f(x+s, y+t) \tag{2}$$

$$a = (m-1)/2 , b = (n-1)/2$$

$$x = 0,1,2,\ldots M-1 , y = 0,1,2,\ldots N-1$$

A complete images after filtering processing can be obtained. In order to extract the texture details information of image, the sum of coefficient of the fractional differential mask is not zero[12]. In order to make fractional differential with better rotation invariant, we also construct fractional differential mask operators of thyroid tumor images, as follows Table1 and Table 2.

Table 1. Fractional differential mask of thyroid tumor ultrasonic image

$(v^2-v)/2$	0	$(v^2-v)/2$	0	$(v^2-v)/2$
0	$-v$	$-v$	$-v$	0
$(v^2-v)/2$	0	8	0	$(v^2-v)/2$
0	$-v$	$-v$	$-v$	0
$(v^2-v)/2$	0	$(v^2-v)/2$	0	$(v^2-v)/2$

Table 2. Fractional differential mask of thyroid tumor radionuclide image

(v4-6v3+11v2-6v)/24	0	$(v^4-6v^3+11v^2-6v)/24$	0	$(v^4-6v^3+11v^2-6v)/24$
0	$(-v^3+3v^2-2v)/6$	$(-v^3+3v^2-2v)/6$	$(-v^3+3v^2-2v)/6$	0
(v4-6v3+11v2-6v)/24	$(v^3+3v^2-2v)/6$	$2(v^2-v)$	-v	1
0	-v	-v	-v	0
1	0	1	0	1

We also adjust the parameter v of fractional differential mask operator with four directions, represented as x , y right diagonal and left diagonal respectively. Ultimately we get the enhancing images after fractional differential processing. As shown in Fig.2.

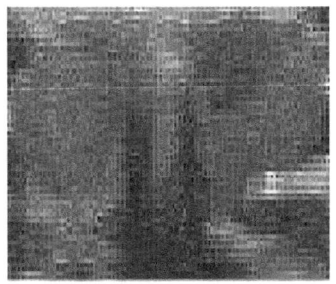   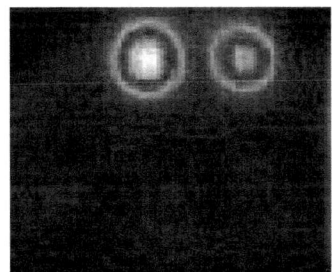

(a) ultrasonic image   (b)radionuclide image

Fig. 2. The image after fractional derivatives processing

4   Normalize Cut Based on Fractional Differential

$G =(V, E, W)$ is used to represent image, V is the set of all the nodes in the graph. E is the set of the edge with connecting the two nodes. W is similarity matrix, composed by the item w_{ij}, w_{ij} represents similarity between the two nodes. Assume that divided graph G into two disjoint subsets A and B, subject to $A \cup B = V$ $A \cap B = \emptyset$. The dissimilarity degree between two subsets =can be expressed as follows.

$$Cut(A, B) = \sum_{\substack{i \in A, j \in B \\ (i, j) \in E}} w_{ij}$$

(3)

The best effect of image segmentation is to make the cut value minimum. Cut value become big with the dividing number of two sides increasing. Assuming the weight value of edges is in inverse proportion to the distance between two points, the division value of outlier is very small. It segments outliers .Ncut put forward a standard division method, as following formula (4).

$$Ncut(A,B) = Cut(A,B)(\frac{1}{Vol(A)} + \frac{1}{Vol(B)}) \qquad (4)$$

$$Vol(A) = assoc(A,V) = \sum_{u \in A, v \in V} w(u,v)$$

$$Vol(B) = assoc(B,V) = \sum_{u \in B, v \in V} w(u,v)$$

According to the thought in [13] and combined with the form of Reyleigh quotient, the rules of Ncut is transformed into solving generalized eigenvalue.

$$(D-W)y = \lambda Dy \qquad (5)$$

There, D is diagonal matrix (diagonal elements is $\sum w_{ij}$), λ , y respectively is eigenvalues and eigenvectors.

According to the type (5), working out Fiedler value and Fiedler vector and combined with the smallest several discrete eigenvectors to segment to get segmentation images[14] . As shown in Fig.3.

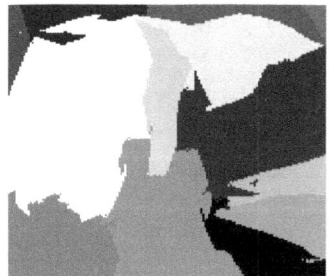   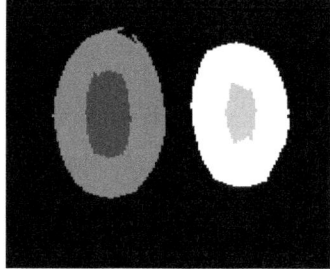

(a) ultrasonic image   (b)radionuclide image

Fig. 3. The segment image to eigenvectors of thyroid tumor

Eigenvectors has good ability with organization distinguished. It distinguishes pixels belonging to the different organizations and owns the similar or identical gray value in the thyroid tumors images. Based on fractional differential method to get edge figures, it together feature space points as the class group corresponding to different regional organizations and the classification results is mapped back into image space.

5 Experimental Results and Analysis

Experimental environment of this paper is Matlab7.1, Dell, CPU2.53 GB, memory 2 GB. In order to verify the feasibility of this method, we simulate and test images, the following is the segmentation results of this paper method about thyroid tumor ultrasonic image and radionuclide image, compared with the segmentation results of the fractional differential method and the segmentation results of the normalized cut method. As shown in Fig.4, Fig5 and Fig.6.

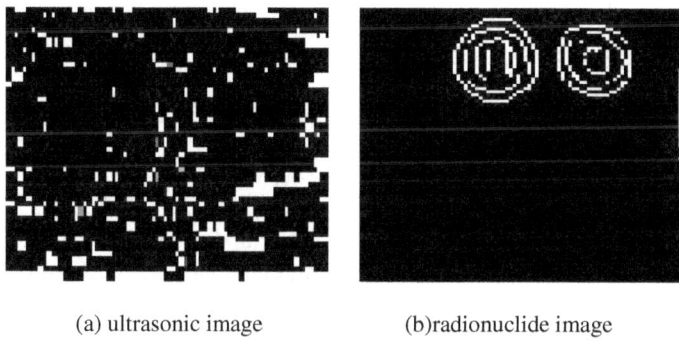

(a) ultrasonic image   (b)radionuclide image

Fig. 4. Result of the fractional differential

Through contrasted with the images of thyroid tumor ultrasonic: Normalized cut segmentation method based on fractional differential accurately segment thyroid tumor in the thyroid tumor ultrasonic image and thyroid organs and trachea can also clearly be divided out. It lets the trachea as the rod of image registration and prepares for registration of the characteristic class. And the normalized cut method results have not segment the thyroid tumor, and do not get the characteristics regions of registration.

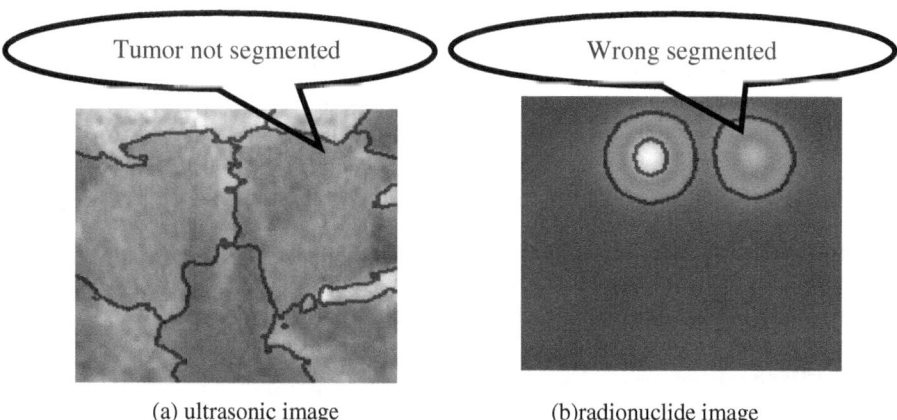

(a) ultrasonic image   (b)radionuclide image

Fig. 5. Result of the normalized cut

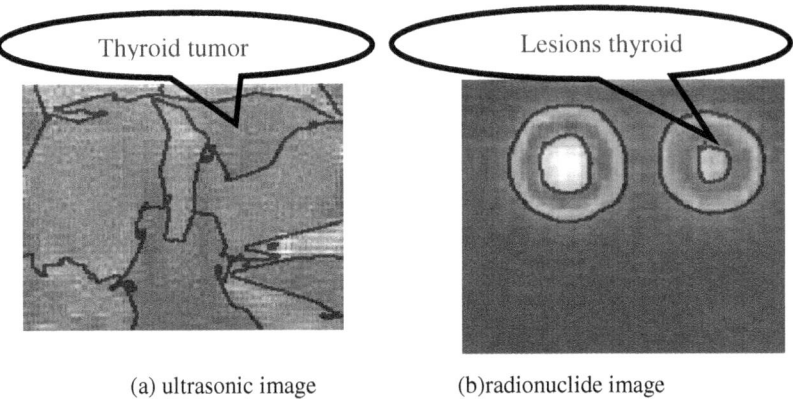

(a) ultrasonic image   (b)radionuclide image

Fig. 6. Result of the improved normalized cut

Through contrasted with the images of thyroid tumor radionuclide: Normalized cut segmentation method based on fractional differential can accurately segment thyroid tumor in the thyroid tumor radionuclide image, the right round is smaller than on the left side of the thyroid in the thyroid radionuclide images. It proves that the thyroid have lesions. So it is possible to achieve registration. And the normalized cut method can segment the thyroid tumor, but it is not accurate enough as registration image.

6   Conclusions and Future Work

Through contrasted with results of the experiment: The method based on fractional differential can't accurately segment the outline of target images. And the proposed normalized cut method   based on the fractional differential can segment the outline of images. The normalized cut algorithm based on the fractional differential is not only used to segment the areas of thyroid tumor images, but also to realize image registration of the characteristic class. So the algorithm is practical and effective.

The next step in research work includes the following aspects: I) features extraction of Ultrasound image and radionuclide image of thyroid tumor; II) feature level registration and fusion of the two different kinds of medical images for thyroid tumor; III) Recognition of thyroid tumor in fusion image.

Acknowledgment. The work is supported by Science Research Program of the Education Department of Hebei Province (2010218) and Open Foundation of Biomedical Multidisciplinary Research Center of Hebei University（BM201103）.

References

1. http://en.wikipedia.org/wiki/Thyroid
2. http://en.wikipedia.org/wiki/Fine-needle_aspiration
3. http://en.wikipedia.org/wiki/Medical_imaging

4. http://www.lw23.com/lunwen_219149237
5. http://en.wikipedia.org/wiki/
   Single-photon_emission_computed_tomography
6. Tian, J., Bao, S.L., Zhou, Q.M.: Medical image processing and analysis, pp. 96–114. Electronic Industry Press (2003)
7. http://www.cs.berkeley.edu/~malik/papers/SM-ncut.pdf
8. Gao, C.B., Zhou, J.L.: Image enhancement based on quaternion fractional directional differentiation. Acta Automatica Sinica 37(2), 150–159 (2010)
9. Li, W., Zhao, H.M.: Rational function approximation for fractional order differential and integral operators. Acta Automatica Sinica 37(8), 999–1005 (2011)
10. Pu, Y.F., Yuan, X., Liao, K., Chen, Z.L., Zhou, J.L.: Five numerical algorithms of frantional calculus applied in modem signal analyzing and processing. Journal of Sichuan University (Engineering Science Edition) 37(5), 118–124 (2005)
11. Pu, Y.F., Wang, W.X.: Fractional differential masks of digital image and their numerical implementation algorithms. Acta Automatica Sinica 33(11), 1128–1135 (2007)
12. VISTA NICTA and RSISE ANU1st Semester, Image Segmentation, Normalized Cuts. Computer Vision and Image Understanding: Theories and Research (2007)
13. Lin, Y., Tian, J.: A survey on medical image segmentation methods. Pattern Recognition and Artificail Inteligence 15(2), 192–204 (2002)
14. Shi, J.B., Malik, J.: Normalized Cuts and Image Segmentation. IEEE Trans. PAMI (2000)

Cellular Neural Networks for Gold Immunochromatographic Strip Image Segmentation

Nianyin Zeng[1,3], Zidong Wang[2], Yurong Li[1,3], and Min Du[3]

[1] College of Electrical Engineering and Automation, Fuzhou University, Fuzhou
350002, P.R. China
nianyin.zeng@gmail.com
[2] Department of Information Systems and Computing, Brunel University, Uxbridge,
Middlesex, UB8 3PH, United Kingdom
Zidong.Wang@brunel.ac.uk
[3] Fujian Key Laboratory of Medical Instrumentation and Pharmaceutical
Technology, Fuzhou 350002, P.R. China

Abstract. Gold immunochromatographic strip assay provides a rapid, simple, single-copy and on-site way to detect the presence or absence of the target analyte. Comparing to the traditional qualitative or semi-quantitative method, a completely quantitative interpretation of the strips can lead to more functional information than the traditional qualitative or semi-quantitative strip assay. This paper aims to develop a method for accurately segmenting the test line and control line of the gold immunochromatographic strip (GICS) image for quantitatively determining the trace concentrations in the specimen. The canny operator as well as the mathematical morphology method is used to detect and extract the GICS reading-window. Then, the test line and control line of the GICS reading-window are segmented by the cellular neural network (CNN) algorithm. It is shown that the CNN offers a robust method for accurately segmenting the test and control lines via adaptively setting the threshold value, and therefore serves as a novel image methodology for the interpretation of GICS.

Keywords: Gold immunochromatographic strip, cellular neural networks, mathematical morphology, canny operator, image segmentation.

1 Introduction

Gold immunochromatographic strip (GICS) assay is a new lateral-flow immunoassay technique that uses a cellulose membrane as the carrier and a colloidal gold-labeled antigen (or antibody) as the tracer. The GICS assay has recently attracted considerable research attention for qualitative and semi-quantitative monitoring in resource-poor or non-laboratory environments. Applications of the GICS assays include tests on pathogens, drugs, hormones and metabolites in biomedical, phytosanitary, veterinary, feed/food and environmental settings.

J. He et al. (Eds.): HIS 2012, LNCS 7231, pp. 110–120, 2012.

It has become clear that the GICS assay has advantages such as ease of use, short analysis time, low cost, high sensitivity, good specificity, and satisfactory stability [1–3]. Owing its attractive properties, the GICS has gained much research interest in the past few years, and the reported results can be generally classified into three categories. The first category is concerned with the improvement of the biochemical properties of the strips via material selection (see e.g. [10, 17]). The second one is about establishing accurate mathematical models for lateral flow immunoassay in order to optimize strip performance for the purpose of quantification (see e.g. [12, 19, 20, 22]). In the third category, the quantitative instrument of lateral flow immunoassay has been developed that has stirred a great deal of research attention (see e.g. [9, 11, 13–16, 18]).

Up to now, most available methods for developing quantitative instruments involve the reflectance photometers for acquiring immunochromatographic strip signals, see e.g. [11, 14, 18]. In this case, mechanical scanning devices are needed which might cause slow operation with bulky style. An alternative way is to develop image-based instruments which are both cost effective and numerically efficient, see e.g. [9, 13, 15, 16]. nevertheless, it is quite challenging to choose a suitable image process technology. In particular, an efficient image segmentation algorithm is of vital importance to the immunochromatographic strip image analysis. In the literature, the Otsu threshold selection method and the fuzzy c-means (FCM) clustering algorithm have been employed to segment the control and test lines of GICS [9, 13, 15]. However, the background in the reading-windows of the GICS image always contains certain level of noises on the strip that might result from the influence of temperature, the humidity as well as the non-uniform penetration of liquid and colloidal gold. For images of low concentration with strong noisy background, it is difficult to infer a threshold because of the possible low signal-noise-ratio (i.e. part of the background intensity is much larger than the signal), which is actually the main drawback of the threshold method and the FCM clustering algorithm [15]. Furthermore, although FCM clustering algorithm has been widely used in the automated image segmentation, it suffers from the local optimum problem and time-consuming computation issue. As such, there is a great need to seek an alternative approach for analyzing the GICS image that aims to avoid the limitations of the aforementioned segmentation techniques while keeping satisfactory accuracies. In search of such an approach, the cellular neural network (CNN) appears to be an ideal candidate for segregating the reading-window from the GICS images extracted by the canny operator and mathematical morphology method.

Cellular Neural Network (CNN), proposed by [4, 5] in 1988, is a large-scale nonlinear analog circuit capable of processing a large amount of information in parallel and in real time. In the past decade, CNNs have gained much attention with wide applications in image and signal processing, robotics and pattern recognition. The general idea of CNN is to combine the architecture of cellular automata with neural networks. It is remarkable that CNN allows for efficient VLSI (very-large-scale integration) implementation of analogue, array-computing structures. Such devices possess a huge processing power that can be

employed to solve numerically expensive problems [21]. Unfortunately, despite
its great application potential, the CNN algorithms have not yet been considered
in GICS image processing, and the main intention of this paper is therefore to
fill the gap by looking into how the CNN algorithms can be exploited to segment
the GICS image by outperforming the traditional FCM clustering algorithm.

It should be pointed out that, the GICS image itself exhibits the following
distinguishing features that add to the difficulties in its processing. First, in
order to improve the efficiency and effectiveness, we only focus on the GICS
reading-windows with the test and control lines appearing on the nitrocellulose
membrane. Thus, it would be better to obtain the reading-window through segmentation. Second, the test and control lines may appear blurred, uncertain, and
mixed with background because they are usually made/smeared by a roller in a
non-uniform way. Furthermore, when the testing liquid (e.g. urine, blood, serum)
is added to the strip, there might be a lot of interference signals appearing on the
strip. With hope to address the above listed challenges, we aim to develop a cellular neural network in combination with the mathematical morphology method
in order to achieve the segmentation of the GICS image. The proposed algorithm
offers a novel image methodology for interpreting gold immunochromatographic
strip.

The rest of this paper is organized as follows. The gold immunochromatographic strip assay is introduced in Section 2. In Section 3, the canny operator
as well as mathematical morphology method for the GICS reading-widow extraction are summarized, and the CNNs for the filtering and segmentation of
GICS reading-window images are described. The results of image segmentation
by the proposed method are discussed in Section 4 and the overall performance
is also demonstrated. Finally, concluding remarks are given in Section 5.

2   The Gold Immunochromatographic Strip Image and Problem Formulation

Gold immunochromatographic strip is based on colloidal gold labeled and chro-
matographic technology (Fig. 1). A typical immunochromatographic strip design
utilizes the specific interaction between antigens and antibodies. In this paper,
we focus on the sandwich format of GICS where one antibody is immobilized
on the nitrocellulose membranes or other solid phase. The other antibody is labeled with colloidal gold. The labeled antibody is dried on a piece of low protein
binding material in conjugate pad. When the specimen passes through and re-
wet the material that is dried with the antibody conjugate, it will release the
antibody conjugate. If the sample contains the antigen to be detected, the antigen will react with antibody conjugate and form an antigen-antibody conjugate
compound. The compound continues to move by capillary action to the membrane where the capture antibody is embedded. The antibody will capture the
antigen-antibody conjugate to form a sandwich type compound. This sandwich
type compound will stay on the membrane and form a visible red or purple red
color band or spot at the test and the control lines, otherwise the redundant
compound goes forward to the absorbent pad.

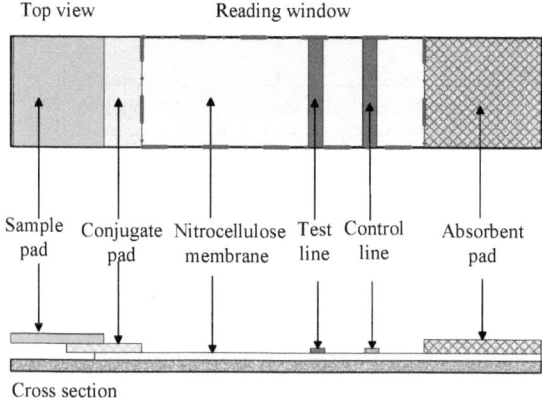

Fig. 1. The schematic structure of the gold immunochromatographic strip

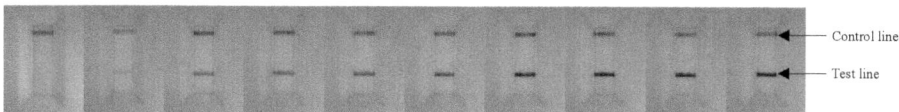

Fig. 2. Images of gold immunochromatographic strip of different concentration(from the left side: 0, 10, 35, 75, 100, 150, 200, 300, 400, 500mIU/ml)

After the antigen-antibody reactions, the red or purple red color caused by the accumulation of the colloidal gold at the test and the control lines will appear on the membrane. Monitoring the strength and area of the red color band provides the basis for the *quantitative* determination of the target molecule. Therefore, the concentration of the measured substance can be determined.

In this study, the gold immunochromatographic strip of human chorionic gonadotropin (hCG) is used as a model. The quantitative tracking result of hCG in serum or urine can provide more useful information in ectopic pregnancy differentiation and in fetal Down syndrome screening test. The GICS images taken from the ten specimens are shown in Fig. 2. The main purpose of this paper is to accurately extract the test line and control line of the GICS images.

3 Process of Gold Immunochromatographic Strip Image

In this section, for the convenience of the readers, we introduce the canny operator as well as mathematical morphology method for the GICS reading window extraction, and then discuss the cellular neural networks for the filtering and segmentation issues of GICS reading-window images described in (Fig. 3).

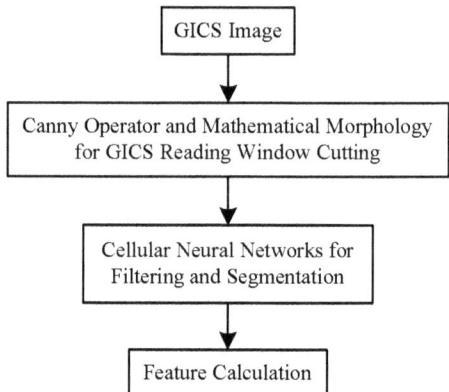

Fig. 3. Image processing for gold immunochromatographic strips

3.1   Canny Operator and Mathematical Morphology for GICS Reading Window Cutting

Canny operator [8] is an excellent edge-detection method which has preferable anti-noise ability. However, the edge got by this method is not a consecutive curve. Thus, after obtaining the edge by canny operator, the mathematical morphology is applied to extract the GICS reading window.

Mathematical morphology is nonlinear image processing methodology that is based on the application of lattice theory to spatial structures [6, 7]. It has become popular in the image processing field due to its rigorous mathematical description and its proven applicability in a number of imaging problems including noise elimination, feature extraction and image compression. The basic operations of mathematical morphology is *erosion* and *dilation*, which are defined as

$$(f \ominus b)(s,t) = max\{f(s+x, t+y) + b(x,y) | (s+x, t+y) \in D_f$$
$$and \ \ (x,y) \in D_b\} \tag{1}$$
$$(f \oplus b)(s,t) = max\{f(s-x, t-y) + b(x,y) | (s-x, t-y) \in D_f$$
$$and \ \ (x,y) \in D_b\} \tag{2}$$

where D_f is the domain of the gray-scale image and D_b is the domain of the structuring element. $\ominus$ and $\oplus$ are expressed as *erosion* and *dilation* operators, respectively. Based on these two operators, the *opening* and the *closing* are defined by

$$f \circ b = (f \ominus b) \oplus b \tag{3}$$
$$f \bullet b = (f \oplus b) \ominus b \tag{4}$$

The *opening* (or *closing*) simplifies by removing the bright (or dark) components that do not fit within the structuring element.

3.2   Cellular Neural Networks

Cellular Neural Network (CNN), proposed in [4, 5] in 1988, is a large-scale non-linear analog circuit which processes signals in real time. The basic circuit unit of cellular neural networks is called a *cell*, see Fig. 4 and Fig. 5. It contains linear and nonlinear circuit elements, which are typically linear capacitors, linear resistors, linear and nonlinear controlled sources, and independent sources. The structure of cellular neural networks is similar to that found in cellular automata; namely, any cell in a cellular neural network is connected only to its neighbor cells. The adjacent cells can interact directly with each other. Cells not directly connected together may affect each other indirectly because of the propagation effects of the continuous-time dynamics of cellular neural networks.

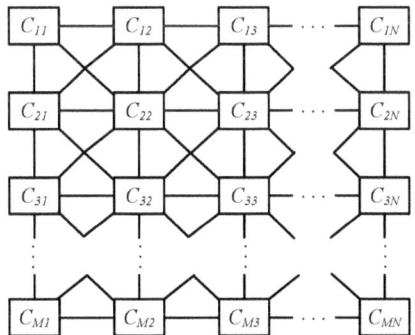

Fig. 4. A two-dimensional cellular neural network

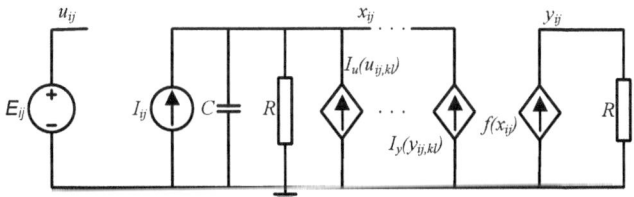

Fig. 5. An example of a *cell* circuit

Consider a two-dimension $M \times N$ cellular neural network shown in Fig. 4, having $M \times N$ cells arranged in M rows and N columns. We denote the *cell* located in the ith row and jth column by C_{ij}. In addition, the *r-neighborhood* (the sphere of influence) in CNN is defined as follows:

$$N_{r(ij)} = \{C_{kl} | max(|k - i|, |l - j|) \le r, 1 \le k \le M, \ 1 \le l \le N\} \tag{5}$$

where r represents the *r-neighborhood* radius of cell C_{ij} and is a positive integral number.

The circuit equations of a cell dynamics are described by the following non-linear ordinary differential equations:

State equation:

$$C\frac{d}{dt}x_{ij}(t) = -\frac{1}{R_x}x_{ij}(t) + \sum_{kl\in N_r} A_{i,j;k,l}y_{kl}(t) + \sum_{kl\in N_r} B_{i,j;k,l}u_{kl}(t) + I_{ij} \quad (6)$$

Output equation:

$$y_{ij}(t) = \frac{1}{2}(|x_{ij}(t) + 1| - |x_{ij}(t) - 1|) \quad (7)$$

Constrained conditions:

$$|x_{ij}(0)| \leq 1, |u_{ij}| \leq 1 \quad (8)$$
$$1 \leq i \leq M, 1 \leq j \leq N \quad (9)$$

where x_{ij}, u_{ij} and y_{ij} are the state, input and output voltages of the specific CNN cell C_{ij}, respectively. The state and output vary in time, the input is static (time-independent), ij refers to grid point associated with a cell on a $2D$ grid, and $kl \in N_r$ is a grid point in the neighborhood within a radius r of the cell C_{ij}. Term $A_{ij,kl}$ represents the linear feedback, $B_{ij,kl}$ is the linear control, while I_{ij} is the cell current (also referred to as bias or threshold) which could be space and time variant. The time constant of a CNN cell is determined by the linear capacitor (C) and the linear resistor (R) and it can be expressed as $\tau = RC$. A CNN cloning template, the program of the CNN array, is given with the linear and nonlinear terms completed by the cell current. Furthermore, a significant theorem for CNN has been given in [5], i.e., if the circuit parameters satisfy

$$A_{ij} > \frac{1}{R}, \quad (10)$$

then

$$\lim_{t\to\infty} |x_{ij}(t)| > 1, \lim_{t\to\infty} |y_{ij}(t)| = \pm 1. \quad (11)$$

The above result guarantees that our cellular neural networks have binary-value outputs. This property is crucial for solving classification problems in image processing applications.

Remark 1. In practice, as the digital image is always of the discrete-time nature, the differential equation of CNN state equation can be rewritten as the difference one when the CNN is applied in the image processing [4]. In general, we let $\tau = 1$ $(R = 1, C = 1)$, so the difference equation of CNN can be seen as follows:

$$x_{ij}(t+1) = \sum_{kl\in N_r} A_{i,j;k,l}y_{kl}(t) + \sum_{kl\in N_r} B_{i,j;k,l}u_{kl}(t) + I_{ij} \quad (12)$$

Thus, we only need to set the feedback template A, control template B and the threshold template I when the CNN is used for image processing.

Remark 2. Generally, the images have different gray-scale range, especially when the target to be segmented is not uniform. Thus, a satisfactory segmentation cannot be achieved by a single threshold value. In this paper, I_{ij} is adaptively changed by the local neighborhood N_r information and can be described as follows:

$$I_{ij} = \frac{MEAN(N_r)}{\max(u)} \tag{13}$$

where $MEAN(N_r)$ represents the average value of the neighborhood N_r information of C_{ij} and $\max(u)$ represents the maximum of the input.

4   Simulation Results and Discussion

4.1   Performance of CNN for Image Segmentation

Considering the image characteristics of the gold immunochromatographic strips, especially when the gray-scales of the test and control lines are different, we divide the extracted reading-window into two parts. One part includes the control line and its background, and another includes the test line and the corresponding background. The threshold template I is set by (13). The feedback template A and control template B of the CNN algorithm in this paper can be described as follows:

$$A = [0 \ 1 \ 0; 1 \ 2 \ 1; 0 \ 1 \ 0] \tag{14}$$

$$B = [0 \ 0.2 \ 0; 0.2 \ 0.2 \ 0.2; 0 \ 0.2 \ 0] \tag{15}$$

In the following, three examples of the segmentation results are shown in Fig. 6, which represent low, middle and high concentration of the specimens respectively.

From Fig. 6, we can see the proposed method can be accurately extracted the test and control lines of the GICS images which obtained by the low, middle and high concentration of hCG in the specimens.

4.2   Feature Calculation

In order to get the quantitative results of the GICS system, a feature parameter should be selected to evaluate the concentration of the specimens. A relative integral optical density (RIOD) [15] based on the Lambert-Beer Law is introduced to acquire the concentration of the measured substance. The RIOD can be described as follows:

$$RIOD = \frac{IOD_T}{IOD_C} = \frac{\sum_{i=1}^{N} \lg \frac{G_0}{G_T{}^i}}{\sum_{j=1}^{M} \lg \frac{G_0}{G_C{}^j}} \tag{16}$$

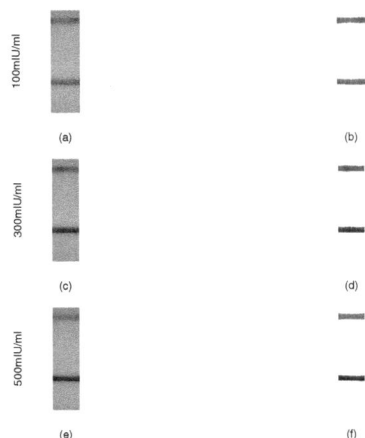

Fig. 6. Three examples of the segmentation results for different concentration of the specimens. Left side: The result of reading-window extraction by canny operator and mathematical morphology; Right side: The result of CNN for image filtering and segmentation.

Table 1. Feature calculation for different concentration specimens

Concentration (mIU/ml)	35	75	100	150	200	300	400	500
RIOD	0.4561	0.6032	0.9028	0.9837	1.8246	2.0095	2.5705	3.4420

where IOD_T and IOD_C represent the reflective integral optical density of the test line and control line, respectively. G_T and G_C are the gray level of pixel in the test line and control line. G_0 is the average gray level of the background in the reading-window.

It is obvious that RIOD can cancel out all the influence, that is, the existence of transmission and scattering will decrease the reflective light intensity, and the non-uniform penetration of water, blood, and colloidal gold will cause the background to only partially reflect the incident light. The results of RIOD for different concentration specimens are given in Table 1. From the Table 1, we can observe a good corresponding relationship between the RIOD and the concentration of hCG. Thus, the proposed method could be a novel image methodology for interpretation of GICS.

5   Conclusions

In this paper, we have presented a novel image methodology for interpretation of gold immunochromatographic strip assay. Specifically, the framework consists of two steps, where the first step is to use the canny operator as well as mathematical morphology method for the GICS reading-window extraction and the second step is to apply cellular neural networks for the GICS reading-window filtering and segmentation. The threshold value of cellular neural networks has been adaptively set according to the local neighborhood information, where the calculated feature parameter corresponds to the concentration of the target in specimen. In conclusion, the proposed approach adds a novel yet effective way for the quantitative interpretation of immunochromatographic strip.

Acknowledgment. This work was supported in part by the International Science and Technology Cooperation Project of China under Grant 2009DFA32050, Natural Science Foundation of China under Grants 61104041, International Science and Technology Cooperation Project of Fujian Province of China under Grant 2009I0016.

References

1. Raphael, C., Harley, Y.: Lateral flow immunoassay. Humana Press (2008)
2. Yager, P., Edwards, T., Fu, E., Helton, K., Nelson, K., Tam, M.R., Weigl, B.H.: Microfuidic diagnostic technologies for global public health. Nature 442, 412–418 (2006)
3. Posthuma-Trumpie, G.A., Korf, J., van Amerongen, A.: Lateral flow (immuno)assay: its strengths, weaknesses, opportunities and threats. A literature survey. Analytical and Bioanalytical Chemistry 393(2), 569–582 (2009)
4. Chua, L.O., Yang, L.: Cellular neural networks: applications. IEEE Transactions on Circuits and Systems 35(10), 1273–1290 (1988)
5. Chua, L.O., Yang, L.: Cellular neural networks: theory. IEEE Transactions on Circuits and Systems 35(10), 1257–1272 (1988)
6. Serra, J.: Image Analysis and Mathematical Morphology. Academic, London (1982)
7. Deng, Z., Yin, Z., Xiong, Y.: High probability impulse noise-removing algorithm based on mathematical morphology. IEEE Signal Processing Letters 14(1), 31–34 (2007)
8. Canny, J.: A computational approach to edge detection. IEEE Transactions on Pattern Analysis and Machine Intelli 8, 679–698 (1986)
9. Chuang, L., Hwang, J., Chang, H., Chang, F., Jong, S.H.: Rapid and simple quantitative measurement of α-fetoprotein by combining immunochromatographic strip test and artificial neural network image analysis system. Clinica. Chimica. Acta. 348, 87–93 (2004)
10. Li, D., Wei, S., Yang, H., Li, Y., Deng, A.: A sensitive immunochromatographic assay using colloidal gold-antibody probe for rapid detection of pharmaceutical indomethacin in water samples. Biosensors and Bioelectronics 24(7), 2277–2280 (2009)
11. Huang, L., Zhang, Y., Xie, C., Qu, J., Huang, H., Wang, X.: Research of reflectance photometer based on optical absorption. International Journal for Light and Electron Optics 121(19), 1725–1728 (2010)
12. Qian, S., Haim, H.: A mathematical model of lateral flow bioreactions applied to sandwich assays. Analytical Biochemistry 322(1), 89–98 (2003)
13. Sumonphan, E., Auephanwiriyakul, S., Theera-Umpon, N.: Interpretation of nevirapine concentration from immunochromatographic strip test using support vector regression. In: Proceedings of 2008 IEEE International Conference on Mechatronics and Automation, pp. 633–637. IEEE Press (2008)

14. Faulstich, K., Gruler, R., Eberhard, M., Haberstroh, K.: Developing rapid mobile POC systems. Part 1:Devices and applications for lateral-flow immunodiagnostics. IVD Technology 13(6), 47–53 (2007)
15. Li, Y., Zeng, N., Du, M.: A novel image methodology for interpretation of gold immunochromatographic strip. Journal of Computers 6(3), 540–547 (2011)
16. Lin, C., Wu, C., Hsu, H., Li, K., Lin, L.: Rapid bio-test strips reader with image processing technology. Optik 115(8), 363–369 (2004)
17. Kaur, J., Singh, K., Boro, R., Thampi, K., Raje, M., Varshney, G.: Immunochromatographic dipstick assay format using gold nanoparticles labeled protein-hapten conjugate for the detection of atrazine. Environmental Science and Technology 41(14), 5028–5036 (2007)
18. Li, J., Ouellette, A., Giovangrandi, L., Cooper, D., Ricco, A., Kovacs, G.: Optical scanner for immunoassays with up-converting phosphorescent labels. IEEE Transactions on Biomedical Engineering 55(5), 1560–1571 (2008)
19. Zeng, N., Wang, Z., Li, Y., Du, M., Liu, X.: Identification of nonlinear lateral flow immunoassay state space models via particle filter approach. IEEE Transactions on Nanotechnology (accepted)
20. Zeng, N., Wang, Z., Li, Y., Du, M., Liu, X.: A hybrid EKF and switching PSO algorithm for joint state and parameter estimation of lateral flow immunoassay models. IEEE/ACM Transactions on Computational Biology and Bioinformatics 9(2), 321–329 (2012)
21. Zineddin, B., Wang, Z., Shi, Y., Li, Y., Du, M., Liu, X.: A multi-view approach to cDNA microarray analysis. International Journal of Computational Biology and Drug Design 3(2), 91–111 (2010)
22. Zeng, N., Wang, Z., Li, Y., Du, M., Liu, X.: Inference of nonlinear state-space models for sandwich-type lateral flow immunoassay using extended Kalman filtering. IEEE Transactions on Biomedical Engineering 58(7), 1959–1966 (2011)

A New Classification Method for Human Gene Splice Site Prediction

Dan Wei[1,2], Weiwei Zhuang[1,2], Qingshan Jiang[2,*], and Yanjie Wei[2]

[1] Cognitive Science Department and Fujian Key Laboratory of the Brain-like Intelligent Systems,
Xiamen University, Xiamen, China
{dan.wei,ww.zhuang}@siat.ac.cn
[2] Shenzhen Institutes of Advanced Technology, Chinese Academy of Sciences, China
{qs.jiang,yj.wei}@siat.ac.cn

Abstract. Human splicing site prediction is important for identifying the complete structure of genes in Human genomes. Machine learning method is capable of distinguishing the different splice sites in genes. For machine learning method, feature extraction is a key step in dealing with the problem of splicing site identification. Encoding schema is a widely used method to encode gene sequences by feature vectors. However, this method ignores the information of the period-3 behavior of the splice sites and sequential information in the sequence. In this paper, a new feature extraction method, based on orthogonal encoding, codon usage and the sequential information, is proposed to map splice site sequences into feature vectors. Classification is performed using a Support Vector Machine (SVM) method. The experimental results show that the new method can predict human splice sites with high classification accuracy.

Keywords: Splice Site, Feature Extraction, SVM.

1 Introduction

With the development of Human Genome Project, an increasingly important task is to analyze genome sequences for the location and structure of their genes. For human genomes, a gene is not a continuous sequence in the DNA, but consists of a set of coding fragments, known as exons, which are separated by non-coding intervening fragments, known as introns [1]. The boundaries between extrons and introns are called splice sites, which are donor splice sites and acceptor splice sites. Accurate prediction of splice sites plays a key role in human genes and genes' structure detection.

Various computational methods have been developed for splice site detection, such as Bayesian networks [2], artificial neural network (ANN) [3-4], discriminant analysis [5-6], support vector machine (SVM) [7-9], and so on. These methods primarily seek consensus motifs or features in the splice sites and the surrounding region by training samples which contain labeled true and false splice sites.

The feature extraction is a key step in classification of splice sites. Two popular methods for feature extraction of splice site prediction are probabilistic model [4] [10-11] and encoding schema [1][9][12]. The probabilistic models, such as the weight

J. He et al. (Eds.): HIS 2012, LNCS 7231, pp. 121–130, 2012.
© Springer-Verlag Berlin Heidelberg 2012

matrix models (WMM) [10] and the weight array model (WAM) [11], are available to model local sequence behavior. WMM uses the nucleotide frequencies at each position, and WAM describes the relationships between adjacent nucleotides by the first order Markov model (MM1). Yet, they require the manual selection of information source [13]. In contrast, Encoding schema such as orthogonal encoding has the advantage of simple process. Orthogonal encoding, in which nucleotides in sequence are viewed as unordered categorical values, is a widely used method to encode DNA sequences by feature vectors. Although orthogonal encoding is effective in many cases, its accuracy may be affected because of ignoring the orders of nucleotides and codon usage. In order to improve the accuracy of splice site prediction, it is necessary to find a more effective feature extraction method to transform splice site sequence to a feature vector.

In this paper, we will apply SVM and a new feature extraction method, which combine orthogonal encoding with codon usage and the sequential information, to the prediction of human splice sites. The rest of this paper is organized as follows. In section 2, we describe splice site prediction problem and related work. Section 3 presents the feature extraction method and the SVM method. Experimental results and analysis are presented in section 4. Finally, section 5 presents our conclusion and discusses directions for future work.

2   Related Work

The exon-intron boundary is called the donor splice site and intron region starts with 'GT' consensus dinucleotide. The intron-exon boundary is called the acceptor splice site and consists of a consensus dinucleotide 'AG' as the last two nucleotides of the intron. The splice site recognition problem is to identify whether a candidate sequence is a splice site or not, and to identify type of splice site, either exon-intron (EI) or intron-exon (IE) [9]. Due to common occurrences of 'GT' or 'AG' consensus dinucleotides at locations other than splice sites of a gene sequence, splicing site prediction is difficult.

Classification based methods have been used to predict splice sites. To use splice site sequence classification analysis, a candidate splice site sequence is represented as a feature vector, and then the classifier takes the feature vectors of training samples as input to train model. Using the obtained training model, the classifier can predict the unknown splice sites. There are two steps in the classification of splice sites:

(1) **Feature extraction:** Good input representations make it easier for the classifier to recognize the underlying regularities. In feature extraction, orthogonal encoding [1][9] is widely used to encode DNA sequences by features vectors. In orthogonal encoding, each nucleotide is represented with 4 binary (0/1) bits. Only one binary variable is set to 1 to represent one of the possible categorical values and the rest are all set to 0. For instance, the nucleotide A can be represented by '1000'. This mapping feature method is simple and allows achieving better classification results than more compact mapping schemes [14]. In order to deal with ambiguous input data, Salekdeh et al. [12] employed a novel

encoding schema, by which only four encoding patterns for ambiguous values are used.

(2) **Classification:** A set of labeled training data is used to train a classifier. The result of training process is a learned model classifier that can separate the categories of sequence samples. Different classification schemes from machine learning are used for this purpose. These classification techniques include artificial neural network (ANN), support vector machine (SVM), etc. These methods learn the complex features of neighborhoods surrounding the consensus dinucleotides 'AG' or 'GT' by a complex non-linear transformation. SVM has gotten wide attention due to its optimal solution, discriminative power and performance, and has been used in splice site detection with high accuracies [7] [15].

For splice site sequences, the exon region exits in upstream of donor and downstream of acceptor, on the other hand, the sequence are ordered by four nucleotides, these will produce some characters as follows:

1) The detection the period-3 behavior of the candidate splice sites can be used for their recognition [16].
2) The codon bias can also be found upstream of most donor and downstream of most acceptor.
3) The sequential relationships enable the inclusion of biological knowledge to differentiate compositional differences of nucleotides in a splice site.

Therefore, codon usage and the sequential relationships between tri-nucleoties are feature information of the exon regions normally exhibiting a period-3 behavior. Whereas, nucleotides in splice sites sequence are viewed as unordered categorical values in encoding method and the information of codon usage is ignored, the information of codon usage and the sequential relationships may be lost, and then the accuracy of encoding method may be affected. In order to solve this problem and improve the accuracy of splice site prediction, we propose a feature extraction method, which combines the orthogonal encoding with the sequential information and codon usage, to represent the splice site sequences, and apply SVM to the prediction of splice sites.

3   The New Method for Splice Site Prediction

We use a new feature extraction method to represent the splice site sequences and then employ SVM to classify the sequences into three classes: EI, IE and false splice site. The process is shown in Figure 1.

In Figure 1, the known samples are labeled splice sties sequences, and the unknown samples are the sequences whose category is unknown. The module of feature extraction maps the original splice site sequences into vectors of real numbers in feature space. Job type distinguishes the input sequence as either training sample or predicting sample. Classification is performed using multiclass SVM.

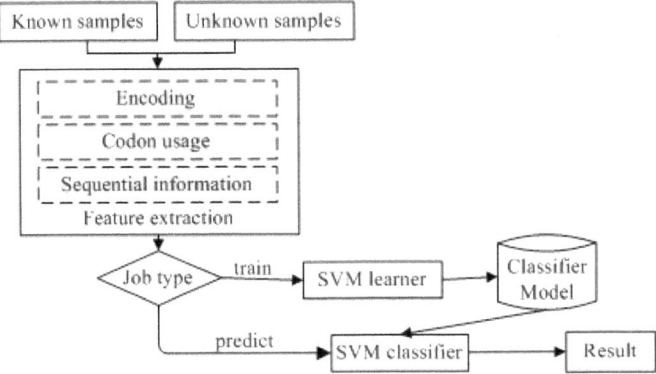

Fig. 1. The flowchart of the splice sites prediction

3.1   Feature Extraction

In order to extract more information in splice site sequences, we use three approaches, orthogonal encoding, codon usage and sequential information, to map the sequence to feature vectors.

3.1.1   Encoding

Orthogonal encoding transforms a splice site sequence with length l into a $4*l$ dimensional number vector. In orthogonal encoding, each nucleotide is represented by a 4 bit number, $A \rightarrow 1000$, $G \rightarrow 0100$, $T \rightarrow 0010$ and $C \rightarrow 0001$.

3.1.2   Codon Usage

There are 64 different codons, therefore each sequence is represented by a vector containing 64 elements. Due to code degeneracy, each amino acid corresponds to 1-6 codons. For instance, the codons of serine are TCT, TCC, TCA, TCG, AGT and AGC. The 64 codons can be divided into 21 classes. In each class, the frequency of codon can be defined,

$$f_{ij} = C_{ij} \Big/ \sum_{j=1}^{n_i} C_{ij} \tag{1}$$

where C_{ij} is the number of occurrences of synonymous codon j of amino acid i and

n_i is the number of synonymous codons encoding amino acid i. The information of codon usage can be represented by a vector $(f_1, f_2, \ldots, f_{64})$.

3.1.3   Sequential Information

In our previous work [17], we extracted the sequential feature using sequence structure and composition for DNA sequence. In order to detect the sequential relationships and the period-3 behavior, we use the sequential feature vector of tri-nucleotides as follows:

(1) Search and locate each tri-nucleotide in a sequence.

(2) w denotes a tri-nucleotide in the sequence. p_r is the location of the rth occurrence of w, where $p_0 = 0$. And α_r can be given as,

$$\alpha_r = \frac{1}{p_r - p_{r-1}} (1 \le r \le m) \qquad (2)$$

in which m stands for the number of occurrences of w in S.

(3) β_j is partial sum of $\{\alpha_r\}$ and calculated by the following formula:

$$\beta_j = \sum_{r=1}^{j} \alpha_r (1 \le j \le m) \qquad (3)$$

(4) Construct a discrete probability distribution $Q = (q_1, q_2, ..., q_m)$, where $q_i = \beta_i / \sum_{i=1}^{m} \beta_i$, and $\sum_{i=1}^{m} q_i = 1$

(5) The *Shannon* entropy of discrete probability distribution is calculated by

$$h = -\sum_{i=1}^{m} q_i \log_2 q_i \qquad (4)$$

These tri-nucleotides in the feature vector are denoted by $(h_1, h_2, ..., h_{64})$, where h_i means the feature representation of the ith tri-nucleotide.

3.1.4 The Algorithm of the Feature Extraction

In order to extract abundant information contained in the splice site sequence and improve the accuracy of prediction, we propose a new feature extraction method, which combine the orthogonal encoding with codon usage and sequential information (ECS), to represent the splice site sequences. The algorithm is outlined as follow:

```
Algorithm ECS
Input: The splice site sequences, S₁,S₂...,S_M, length of se-
quence, l
Output: Feature vectors
Begin
   For i=1 to M, Do
   Mapping Sᵢ into a vector, (e₁,e₂,...,e₄ₗ), of binary(0/1)
   variables according to orthogonal encoding schema;
   Search and locate each tri-nucleotide in Sᵢ;
   For tri-nucleotides in Sᵢ, use Eqn. (1) to calculate
   and construct the vector, (f₁,f₂,...,f₆₄);
   For tri-nucleotides in Sᵢ, calculate and construct the
   vector, (h₁,h₂,...,h₆₄), according to Eqn. (2)-(4);
End For
```

Merge three vectors, $(e_1, e_2, \ldots, e_{4 \cdot l})$, $(f_1, f_2, \ldots, f_{64})$ and
$(h_1, h_2, \ldots, h_{64})$, as a combining vector $(v_1, v_2, \ldots, v_{4 \cdot l + 128})$;
    Return the vector, $(v_1, v_2, \ldots, v_{4 \cdot l + 128})$;
End.

3.2   Support Vector Machine (SVM)

The goal of SVM [18] is to design classifier f: X->Y, which minimizes probability of misclassification.

$$R(f) = \int L(y, f(x)) dP(x, y) \tag{5}$$

where L(y, f(x)) is 1/0-loss function: L(y, f(x)) = 0 if y = f(x) or L(y, f(x)) = 1 if y ≠ f(x). An independently labeled training set {(x$_1$, y$_1$), ..., (x$_n$, y$_n$)} generated by unknown probability distribution P(x, y) is available. The Statistical Learning Theory introduces upper bounds on the expected risk R. For the linear functions, the upper bound can be efficiently minimized through maximization of margin. Linear classifier f(x) = argmax fk(x) uses linear discriminant functions:

$$f_k(x) = w_k^T \cdot x + b_k, k \in y \tag{6}$$

Learning of the linear multi-class SVM corresponds to solving the Quadratic Programming problem (primal SVM QP problem):

$$(w_k, b_k, k \in y) = \arg\min_{w_k, b_k, \varepsilon_i^k} \frac{1}{2} \sum_{k \in y} \|w_k\|^2 + C \cdot \sum_{i \in I, k \in y \setminus \{y_i\}} \varepsilon_i^k \tag{7}$$

subject to

$$w_{y_i}^T \cdot x_i + b_{y_i} - (w_k^T \cdot x_i + b_k) \geq 1 - \varepsilon_i^k \tag{8}$$

where $\varepsilon_i^k \geq 0, i \in I, k \in y \setminus \{y_i\}$.

Training data should be correctly classified, and the set of inequalities $f_{y_i}(x_i) - f_k(x_i) > \varepsilon, k \neq y_i$ holds. Slack variables ε_i^k allow coping with non-separable data by relaxing the constraints. Minimization of $\sum \|w_k\|^2$ leads to maximization of margin, and minimization of $\sum \varepsilon_i^k$ leads to minimization of number of overlapping patterns.

4   Experiments and Result Analysis

To illustrate the effectiveness of our new feature extraction approach, we apply the approach on real human splice site sequences, which are taken from HS3D (Homo Sapiens Splice Sites Data set) [19]. All the experimental studies are conducted under the environment of Windows XP operating system running on Intel P4 1.83 GHz CPU with 2 GB of RAM.

4.1   Data Set

HS3D, which is downloaded from http://www.sci.unisannio.it/docenti/rampone/. includes introns, exons and splice site sequences extracted from GeneBank Rel.123. The splice site sequences in HS3D are with length of 140 nucleotides. There are 2796 true donor sites and 2880 true acceptor sites, and 271 937 false donor sites and 329 374 false acceptor sites. Each sequence in HS3D consists of 140 nucleotides surrounding a candidate splice site. In our experiments, we take all the true donor and acceptor sites and randomly select equal number of false sites, the description of the data set is shown in Table 1.

Table 1. Summary of Splice Site Training and Test Data Sets

Splice sites Categories	Number of Splice Site Sequences	
	Training Set	**Test Set**
EI	2237	559
IE	2304	576
False	4541	1135

The exon-intron boundaries (EI) are characterized by the consensus dinucleotide 'GT', and the intron-exon boundaries (IE) are characterized by the consensus dinucleotide 'AG'. Gene sequence also may contain false splice site sequences, which have 'AG' or 'GT' dinucleotide, but they do not correspond to known splice sites. The sequences, which contain consensus dinucleotide 'AG' or 'GT' dinucleotide and do not correspond to known splice sites, are regarded as false splice sites.

4.2   Evaluation

To measure the quality of the prediction results, the experiments use   sensitivity (S_N), specificity (S_P), and accuracy (Acc) to evaluate the clustering performance.

$$S_N = TP/(TP + FN) \tag{9}$$

$$S_P = TN/(TN + FP) \tag{10}$$

$$Acc = (S_N + S_P)/2 \tag{11}$$

where TP, FN, TN, and FP represent the number of true positives, false negatives, true negatives and false positives, respectively.

4.3   Classification Results

In our experiments, the multiclass SVM classifier is tested using a five-fold cross-validation to estimate the accuracy of classification.

We evaluate the effectiveness of different feature extraction methods including Encoding, combining Encoding with codon usage (EC), combining encoding with sequential information (ES), as well as combining encoding with codon usage and sequential information (ECS) method, for splice site classification. Experimental results are shown in Table 2 and Table 3, respectively.

Table 2. Performance of the four feature extraction methods using SVM on exon-intron boundaries (EI)

Feature	Sp	Sn	Acc
Encoding	0.906	0.902	0.904
EC	0.946	0.910	0.928
ES	0.951	0.913	0.932
ECS	**0.977**	**0.918**	**0.948**

Table 3. Performance of the four feature extraction methods using SVM on intron-exon boundaries (IE)

Feature	Sp	Sn	Acc
Encoding	0.909	0.893	0.901
EC	0.930	0.906	0.918
ES	0.938	0.908	0.923
ECS	**0.962**	**0.912**	**0.937**

From table 2 and Table 3, we observe that the S_P and S_n are increased after adding codon usage or sequential information of tri-nucleotide to encoding feature, this may be due to the information of codon usage or period-3 behavior of the candidate splice site sequences. When we consider both the codon usage and sequential features in the ECS method, a higher accuracy rate is obtained, and this shows ECS outperforms all the other methods both in prediction exon-intron sites and intron-exon sites.

We also compare our proposed method, a combination of ECS with SVM (ECS_SVM), with other methods, including the first order weight matrix model (WMM1) based on BPNN and RBFN [4], and the first order Markov model (MM1) based on BPNN and RBFN [4]. Table 4 shows the performance of these five methods.

Table 4. Accuracies produced by ECS_SVM and other methods

Splice sites Categories	WMM1-BPNN	WMM1-RBFN	MM1-BPNN	MM1-RBFN	ECS_SVM
EI	0.895	0.893	0.927	0.930	**0.948**
IE	0.880	0.878	0.925	0.921	**0.937**

Results show that our method, ECS_SVM, outperforms other detection methods, such as WMM1-BPNN, WMM1-RBFN, MM1-BPNN, and MM1-RBFN, both in detection exon-intron sites and intron-exon sites.

5   Conclusions and Future Work

In this paper, we presented a new method that can identify human acceptor and donor splice sites. Combining orthogonal encoding with the sequential information and codon usage, the new method captures the sequence information and helps to achieve better results for human splice site prediction. Future work includes studying other features of splice sites and developing an effective classification algorithm to improve the accuracy of prediction.

Acknowledgments. This work is supported by the Shenzhen New Industry Development Fund under grant No.CXB201005250021A, the National Natural Science Foundation of China (No.61175123).

References

1. Lorena, A., de Carvalho, A.: Human Splice Site Identification with Multiclass Support Vector Machines and Bagging. In: Kaynak, O., Alpaydın, E., Oja, E., Xu, L. (eds.) ICANN 2003 and ICONIP 2003. LNCS, vol. 2714, pp. 234–241. Springer, Heidelberg (2003)
2. Chen, T.M., Lu, C.C., Li, W.H.: Prediction of splice sites with dependency graphs and their expanded Bayesian networks. Bioinformatics 21(4), 471–482 (2005)
3. Ho, L.S., Rajapakse, J.C.: Splice site detection with a higher-order Markov model implemented on a neural network. Genome Informatics 14, 64–72 (2003)
4. Baten, A.K.M.A., Halgamuge, S.K., Chang, B., Wickramarachchi, N.: Biological sequence data preprocessing for classification: A case study in splice site identification. In: Proceedings 4th International Symposium on Neural Networks Advances in Neural Networks, vol. 2, pp. 1221–1230 (2007)
5. Chuang, J.S., Roth, D.: Splice site prediction using a sparse network of winnows. Technical Report, University of Illinois, Urbana-Champaign (2001)
6. Zhang, L.R., Luo, L.F.: Splice site prediction with quadratic discriminant analysis using diversity measure. Nucleic Acids Research 31(21), 6214–6220 (2003)
7. Sonnenburg, S., Schweikert, G., Philips, P., Behr, J., Ratsch, G.: Accurate splice site prediction using support vector machines. BMC Bioinformatics 8(suppl.), S7 (2007)
8. Varadwaj, P., Purohit, N., Arora, B.: Detection of Splice Sites Using Support Vector Machine. Communications in Computer and Information Science 40(Part 10), 493–502 (2009)
9. Damasevicius, R.: Structural analysis of regulatory DNA sequences using grammar inference and support vector machine. Neurocomputing 73(4-6), 633–638 (2010)
10. Staden, R.: Computer methods to locate signals in nucleic acid sequences. Nucleic Acids Research 12, 505–519 (1984)
11. Zhang, M.Q., Marr, T.G.: A weight array method for splicing signal analysis. Comput. Appl. Biosci. 9, 499–509 (1993)
12. Salekden, A.Y., Wiese, K.C.: Improving Splice-Junctions Classification employing a Novel Encoding Schema and Decision-Tree. In: IEEE Congress on Evolutionary Computation (CEC), New Orleans, LA, June 5-8, pp. 1302–1307 (2011)
13. Degroeve, S., De Baets, B., Van de Peer, Y., Rouzé, P.: Feature subset selection for splice site prediction. Bioinformatics 18(suppl. 2), S75-S83 (2002)

14. Damasevicius, R.: Analysis of binary feature mapping rules for promoter recognition in imbalanced DNA sequence datasets using support vector machine. In: Proceedings of 4th IEEE International Conference on Intelligent Systems, pp. 1120–1125. IEEE Press, Piscataway (2008)
15. Dror, G., Sorek, R., Shamir, R.: Accurate identification of alternatively spliced exons using support vector machine. Bioinformatics 21(7), 897–901 (2005)
16. Akhtar, M.: Comparison of gene and exon prediction techniques for detection of short coding regions, Special Issue on Bioinformatics and Biomedical Systems. International Journal of Information Technology 11(8), 26–35 (2005)
17. Wei, D., Jiang, Q.: A DNA Sequence Distance Measure Approach for Phylogenetic Tree Construction. In: 5th IEEE International Conference on Bio-Inspired Computing: Theories and Applications, pp. 204–212 (2010)
18. Vapnik, V.N.: Statistical Learning Theory. John Wiley, Sons, New York (1998) ISBN: 0471030031
19. Pollastro, P., Rampone, S.: HS3D-Homo Sapiens Splice Sites Dataset. Nucleic Acids Research 2003 Annual Database Issue (2003)

An Association Rule Analysis Framework for Complex Physiological and Genetic Data

Jing He[1], Yanchun Zhang[1], Guangyan Huang[1], Yefei Xin[1], Xiaohui Liu[2],
Hao Lan Zhang[3], Stanley Chiang[4], and Hailun Zhang[5]

[1] Victoria University, Melbourne, Australia
{jing.he,yanchun.zhang,guangyan.huang}@vu.edu.au,
yefei.xin@live.vu.edu.au
[2] Brunel University, UK
xiaohui.liu@brunel.ac.uk
[3] NIT, Zhejiang University, China
haolan.zhang@nit.zju.edu.cn
[4] TLC Medical PTY LTD, Australia
tlcscchiang@hotmail.com
[5]Step High Technology Co Ltd
Hailan.zhangzh@gmail.com

Abstract. Physiological and genetic information has been critical to the successful diagnosis and prognosis of complex diseases. In this paper, we introduce a support-confidence-correlation framework to accurately discover truly meaningful and interesting association rules between complex physiological and genetic data for disease factor analysis, such as type II diabetes (T2DM). We propose a novel Multivariate and Multidimensional Association Rule mining system based on Change Detection (MMARCD). Given a complex data set u_i (e.g. u_1 numerical data streams, u_2 images, u_3 videos, u_4 DNA/RNA sequences) observed at each time tick t, MMARCD incrementally finds correlations and hidden variables that summarise the key relationships across the entire system. Based upon MMARCD, we are able to construct a correlation network for human diseases.

1 Introduction

Over the past two decades, genetic and physiological information has been essential to the diagnosis, prognosis and epidemiological analysis of complex diseases. The availability of comprehensive, aggregated knowledge is crucial to the success of health informatics/bioinformatics in understanding complex diseases; in particular, technologies like DNA/RNA sequencing and physiological mapping have made previously tedious and expensive processes cheaper and easier. In addition, extracting useful knowledge quickens data collection, analysis and distribution.

The existing medical information systems store voluminous and detailed genetic data (e.g. DNA/RNA sequences) and physiological data (e.g. blood pressure and temperature) that may be continuous, sequential, binary or categorical measurements

J. He et al. (Eds.): HIS 2012, LNCS 7231, pp. 131–142, 2012.

recorded at different intervals across life span to monitor the development of complex diseases. Moreover, many complex diseases (or a group of symptoms) such as type II diabetes (T2DM) involve genes with clinical phenotypes [1], raising a new technical challenge in discovering the genotypes underlying human phenotypes.

To cure or alleviate complex diseases, it is critical to identify disease factors that may be associated with observable physical or biochemical characteristics. Traditional statistical approaches like genome-wide association analysis [1] can narrow the set of potentially important linkages between phenotypes and genotypes, but many rules generated are still not interesting to the human disease research. More efficient computer-aided methods are highly demanded for comprehensive analysis of physiological and genetic data.

In this paper, we employ a support-confidence-correlation framework to accurately discover truly meaningful and interesting association rules for disease factor analysis. We propose a novel approach, Multivariate and Multidimensional Association Rule mining system based on Change Detection (MMARCD), of mining multivariate and multidimensional association and correlation rules by using discretisation of change attributes in very large databases of discrete and continuous data. We focus on general association rule mining problems for complex combined physiological and genetic datasets. By utilising advanced data mining techniques [2], MMARCD discovers correlation and association relationships between genetic and physiological data and thereby identify factors that undetectable using current state-of-the-art methods. Furthermore, based on MMARCD, a correlation network for human diseases can be constructed, which handles complex input data, like images, text, video, and stream data. It leads to an appreciation of the effects of genetic mutations and physiological trends in virtually all disorders, and provides the opportunity to study human diseases dynamically.

The rest of the paper is organized as follows. Section 2 presents the related works in genome association and data mining areas. Section 3 details the proposed solution. Section 4 illustrates the expected results. Section 5 concludes this paper and directs future works.

2   Related Works

Many large-scale efforts – in the United States, the United Kingdom, Japan and elsewhere – aim to uncover genetic effects and gene-environment interactions relevant to disease [6, 7, 8, 9, 10, 11]. However, conducting separate association analysis of genetic and physiological observations cannot achieve accurate results, since multiple genetic mutations have frequently been identified in the multiple dimensions. Also, univariate genetic mutations can explain some of the clinical variability observed in single-gene diseases, but usually not all; the residual is probably due to modifier genes and environmental contributors [1]. Identifying the relationship between such modifiers and contributors is a principal challenge, closely allied with the association and correlation analysis for complex genetic and physiological data.

A genome-wide association study (GWA study, or GWAS) also known as a whole genome association study (WGA study, or WGAS) [3, 4, 5, 9, 10, 11], is an examination of genomes of individuals to see if any variant is associated with a disease trait. Typically, single-nucleotide polymorphisms (SNPs) and traits such as major diseases are investigated. GWASs contribute to our understanding of diseases to which there is a genetic predisposition, including genes associated with age-related macular degeneration [12], myocardial infraction, and abnormal cardiac repolarisation intervals [13]. For example, over 1,200 human GWASs have examined over 200 diseases and traits and found almost 4,000 SNP associations [13]. However, not all common and complex diseases have only one or a few common variants as contributing factors. In these cases, the GWA approach would be ineffective since there is no common mutation tagged by a particular gene.

In data mining fields, association rules analysis [12, 13, 14, 15, 16, 17, 18] has been developed over years, but cannot account for cumulative effects. Since the change set of real-world genetics and physiological dataset will be measured as quantitative attributes, the current solutions for association analysis based on quantitative attributes are not adequate [14, 15, 16, 17, 18, 21]. Most related work, including the change coupling detection [19, 20], can only capture change relations among co-changing artifacts within a single change set [19]; it fails to capture change relations that have a consequentiality spread over an interval of time and within multiple change sets.

A network of disorder and disease genes linked by known disorder-gene associations [22] is used to explore all known phenotypes and disease gene associations in a single graph theoretic framework. However, while the current technique supports clinicians and medical researchers to share commonalities in etiology or pathology [22, 23, 24] in the bipartite graph, it cannot deal with the input of complex data like images, text, video, and stream data.

3   Proposed Solution

The system framework is shown in Fig. 1. The following 13 time series including genetic and physiological variables are input into the system:

- Four DNA/RNA sequence (1) – (4): TCF7L2, PPARG, FTO, KCNJ11;
- Eight physiological time series (5) – (12): Number of times pregnant, Plasma glucose concentrations at 2hrs in an oral glucose tolerance test (mg/dL), Diastolic blood pressure (mm Hg), Triceps skinfold thickness (mm), 2-hr serum insulin (mu U/ml), Body mass index, Diabetes pedigree function, Age (years);
- Retinal image (13).

Based upon the above data variables, we start by analysing simple disease (a), genes (b), and physiological observations (c) network separately (Fig. 4). After the association analysis, we are able to produce the correlation complex disease network (Fig. 5).

The detailed algorithm is shown as follows:

```
Collect Genetic and Physiological Time Series Data
Measure and mine the genetic variation (GV)
Measure and mine the physiological changes (PC)
  Measure and mine changes over time-series data
  Measure and mine changes over image data
Calculate anomalous score
Detect the noise and outlier
Link GV and PC and analyse the correlation
Construct correlation disease network
```

The initial data collection for training methods and benchmark data for comparison are obtained from open source databases such as the Cancer Genetic Makers of Susceptibility Project, National Cancer Institute, U.S.A. [6], and National Human Genome Research Institute [7], especially the T2DM data from the Diabetes Genetics Initiative [8].

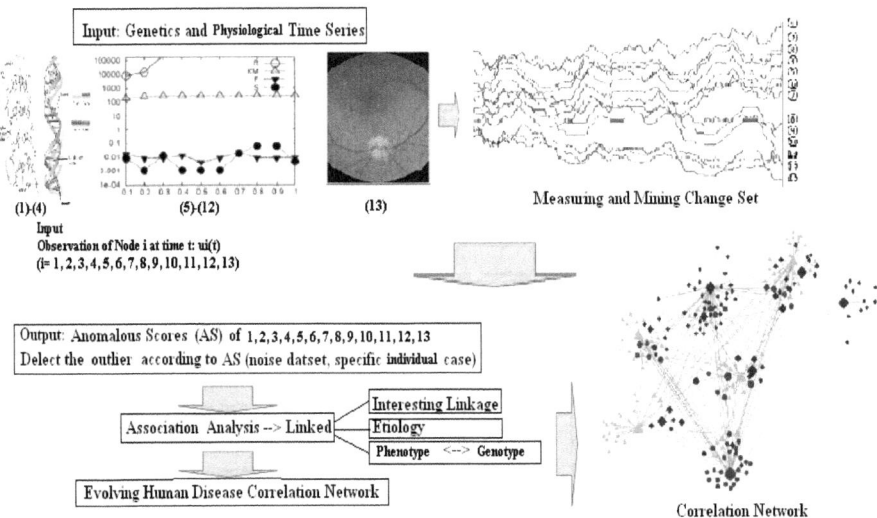

Fig. 1. Problem setting and system framework

The real-world genetic and physiological data are generated at different labs and by different methods. DNA sequence data (from BGI – Large scale genome sequencing research centre) and physiological data (from TLC Medical) will be collected from healthy and diseased tissues. In previous tests and collaborations, BGI supplied 50 Asian patients' DNA/RNA sequences and TLC supplied 200 Australian patients' physiological data. BGI produced DNA sequencing data from cells containing DNA in body fluids (such as blood and saliva), cheek swabs, hairs with follicular tissue at the root, soft bones (such as rib bones), and deep muscle tissue; TCL received medical records for patients with T2DM in a town in north-western Victoria, and some patients are with the kinship relation. In order to handle integration and cleaning of our complex data, we firstly implement a semantic integration as a prelude to the cross-site analysis of genetic [28] and physiological data. The bio-ontology and medical ontology are combined and improved to find correct linkages among medical records with physiological data, the research literature and the associated biological entities for data integration and linkage.

DNA and protein sequences are long chains of chemical components. These components or "building blocks" are four nucleotides (also called bases), namely adenine (A), cytosine (C), guanine (G), and thymine (T). A gene is typically composed of hundreds of individual nucleotides arranged in a particular order. Genetic Variation (GV) is changes in a genomic sequence and is important because it provides the "raw material" for natural selection. A novel aggregate mutation score method based on a data-mining approach of a multiple sequence alignment tool [2] is used to analyse DNA/RNA sequences from over 150 patients to identify novel factors implicated in the pathology of T2DM. The details are: (i) establish a quantitative diagnostic score as an evidence-based improvement on the existing pathological diagnostic criteria. It aligns existing biomarkers such as TCF7L2, PPARG, FTO, KCNJ11 in DNA/RNA sequences to monitor the DNA/RNA mutations and detect common patterns within two groups; (ii) develop an aggregate mutation score based on a multiple sequence alignment tool to identify the differences between the DNA/RNA sequences from healthy tissues (P1) and diseased tissues (P2) related to T2DM. Sequences occurring more frequently in P2 may indicate the genetic factors of T2DM, and those occurring more frequently in P1 may indicate the mechanisms that protect the body from T2DM. Mining the genetic variation is different from mining physiological data because the DNA sequence is non-numeric. Traditional molecular physiological methods do not consider the interconnections between nucleotides, which play an important role in biologic function. Therefore, we fold DNA sequences into three-dimensional structures and the aggregate mutation score calculated based on the interacting structures and the distances between them.

The standard methods of testing for T2DM are the fasting plasma glucose test and oral glucose tolerance test, both of which measure fasting glucose level in the blood; body mass index and blood pressure are also important. For example, microvasculature complications in the eye can be measured to detect the early signs of eye blur. We focus on mining the physiological changes through time-series data and retinal images.

Most of the physiological data, such as blood tests for two-hour glucose and fasting glucose, weight and blood pressure are typical time-series data. The time-series datasets related to T2DM consist of sequences of mostly numerical values or events obtained from repeated measurements over time (e.g. hourly, daily, weekly). Various time-series data mining approaches can be applied to mine such data, including Hoeffding Tree, Very Fast Decision Tree, Concept-adapting Very Fast Decision Tree [32]. We use Euclidean distance between the time-series datasets to measure the change among them according to our previous experiments [25, 26, 29, 30, 31].

Retinal images are important in detection of early stage diabetes; they are used to compare the states of retinal blood vessels. We can develop a new module for automated screening for T2DM retinopathic complications and detect and measure the changes in retinal images. Based on our previous work on automatically generation abstractions of images [26, 27], the proposed data mining system can automatically generate two-dimensional colour images of segments of blood vessels in retina. Through using the DBSCAN, this system can extract the ridges of images that coincide with the vessel centrelines [26, 27]. The ridges can be used to compose primitives in the form of line elements; an image is partitioned into frame for its corresponding patch. For every pixel, the distance feature vectors can be computed to measure the similarity and difference between two images. The feature vector can be further classified using DBSCAN cluster [26, 27] and sequential forward feature selection. This method has been tested on a database and achieved more than 85% accuracy for abnormal blood vessel detection, providing that blood vessels can be effectively detected by applying our method to retinal images. The similarity degree distance based on feature vectors can be applied to measure changes between retinal images.

Based upon the above pre-processing work, all the original DNA/RNA sequence and physiological data has been transferred into the change set as Aggregate Mutation Score, Euclidean Distance, and Similarity Degree Distance.   The noise or outlier can be detected by (i) constructing quantitative representing features of each change set from the same input based on Eigen equation compression, and (ii) calculating the incremental anomalous score based on learning the probability distribution of the quantities. Once the anomalous score surpass the threshold, the corresponding dataset can be considered as noise/outlier. Our previous experiments with finance data and an Intensive Care Unit (ICU) stream dataset proved the efficiency and accuracy of these methods [25].

A single dimension association rule analysis in genetic variation or physiological changes is also performed. If we treat the DNA sequence as the set of items available in the database, then each item has a Boolean variable representing the presence or absence of that item. A Boolean vector of values assigned to these variables can then represent each event. The Boolean vectors can be analysed for event patterns that reflect DNA sequences frequently associated or co-occurring with T2DM. For example, the system can mine association rules formatted as follows, where X is a variable representing a DNA sequence, and GV means genetic variation represented by Aggregate Mutation Score.

GV (X, "30 ... 39") $\Rightarrow$ Disease (X, "T2DM") [support = 2%, confidencee = 60%] (I)

Rule (I) indicates that there is a strong association rule between GV and disease T2DM. A support of 2% for Rule (I) means that 2% of all the DNA sequences under analysis show that certain genetic variations in DNA sequence and diseased DNA sequence are happening together. A confidence value of 60% means that 60% of the DNA sequences, which have the genetic variation, also have T2DM-disease sequence. In this case, if the specific threshold is met, this mined rule indicates that if certain genetic variation (often represented by the Aggregate Mutation Score) falls in the interval "30 – 39", there is a high probability that T2DM will occur. Meanwhile, if the support and confidence surpass the threshold, a link between the DNA sequence and T2DM will be placed. Another example is given by:

$$GV\ (Y,\ ">= 0.5")\Rightarrow Disease\ (Y,\ "T2DM")\ [support = 6\%,\ confidence = 75\%]\quad (II)$$

where Y indicates patients' physiological datasets.

If the specific threshold is met, Rule (II) indicates that if a certain physiological change degree (often represented by the similarity measurement) is more than 0.5 (e.g. physiological indicators of T2DM increase or decrease by 50%), there is high probability that T2DM will occur.

We develop a novel mining multidimensional association rule algorithm to find the strong association rules among GV, PC, and T2DM. The following rules apply:

$$GV\ (P, "30 - 39")\ \wedge\ PC\ (P, " >= 0.5")\Rightarrow Disease\ (P, "T2DM")\qquad\qquad (III)$$

$$GV\ (P, "10 - 25")\ \vee\ PC\ (P, " >= 0.3")\Rightarrow Disease\ (P, "T2DM")\qquad\qquad (IV)$$

$$GV\ (P,\ "30 - 39")\ \wedge\ Disease\ (P,\ "T2DM")\Rightarrow PC\ (P,\ "\geq 0.5")\ \wedge\ Disease\ (P,\ "T2DM")$$
$$(V)$$

Rule (III) indicates both certain GV and PC can cause T2DM and Rule (IV) indicates either certain GV or PC can cause T2DM. Rule (III) and (IV) can be used to identify the risk due to phenotype and genotype factors. Rule (V) indicates GV and PC have a strong relationship, which proves that a genetic mutation can cause change in the physiological condition of patients. We use Rule (III) as an example to explain the association rule discovery process as follows:

Rule (III) is a typical two-dimensional quantitative association rule (see Fig. 2) and a 2D grid to display Rule (III) is shown in Fig. 3, with two quantitative on the left-handed side of the rule and one categorical attribute on the right-handed side of the rule. Rule (III) can be rewritten as:

$$A\_quan1\ \wedge\ A\_quan2\Rightarrow A\_cat\qquad\qquad (VI)$$

where A_quan1 and A_quan2 are two quantitative attributes set on GV and PC such as the Aggregated Mutation Score, Euclidean Distance and Similarity Degree Distance, and A_cat is categorical attributes non-T2DM and T2DM.

Furthermore, a correlation measure will be added to the support-confidence framework for association rule to detect truly meaningful and interesting patterns. Hence, associations can be further analysed to uncover correlation rules, which convey statistical correlations between item sets GV ∧ PC ⇒ T2DM [support, confidence]. This leads to correlation rules of the form GV ∧ PC ⇒ T2DM [support, confidence, correlation]. The classic multivariate association measurement such as $X^2, Lift,$ AllConf, Coherence, Cosine, Kulczynski [32] can be employed and tested; our previous experiments show that both AllConf and Cosine [2] are good correlation measures for large genetic and physiological applications.

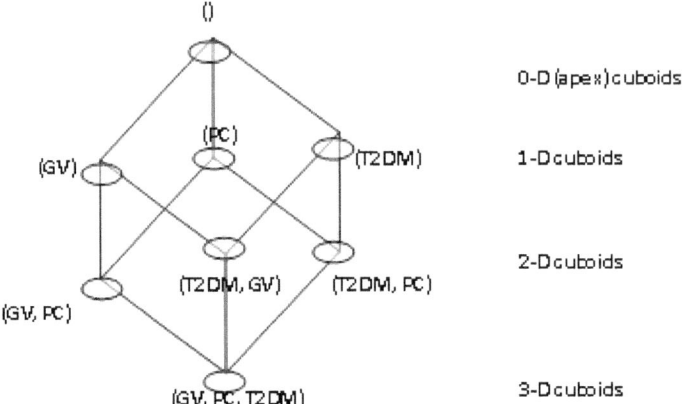

Fig. 2. Lattice of cuboids, making up a 3D cube. The base of the cuboid contains the two dimensions GV and PC and the task-relevant data T2DM.

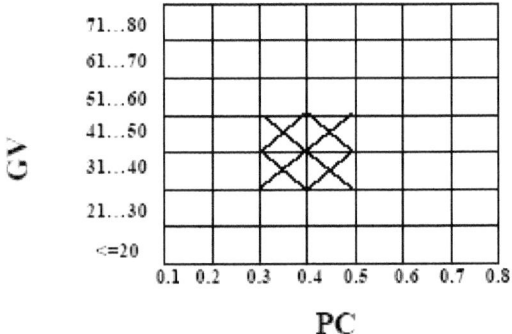

Fig. 3. A 2D grid for tuples representing patients who have high probability of T2DM

4   Expected Results

Based on the single dimension association analysis, we can build the network for disease, gene, and physiological observations separately shown in Fig. 4, which is a snapshot of a single level T2DM network that is a subset of the human disease network where circles, diamonds and rectangles correspond to disease (a), genes (b), and physiological observations (c) respectively. A link is placed to represent the occurrence of the different nodes. For example, in Fig. 4(b), the genes are linked due to the occurrence of the disorder being related with T2DM and is based on the association analysis GV $\Rightarrow$ T2DM (I). Fig. 4(a) is a subset Human Disease Network and the detected T2DM disease relationship is in Sladek's work [10]. Fig. 4(c) is a T2DM Disease Network based on physiological observations and it is based on association analysis PC $\Rightarrow$ T2DM (II).

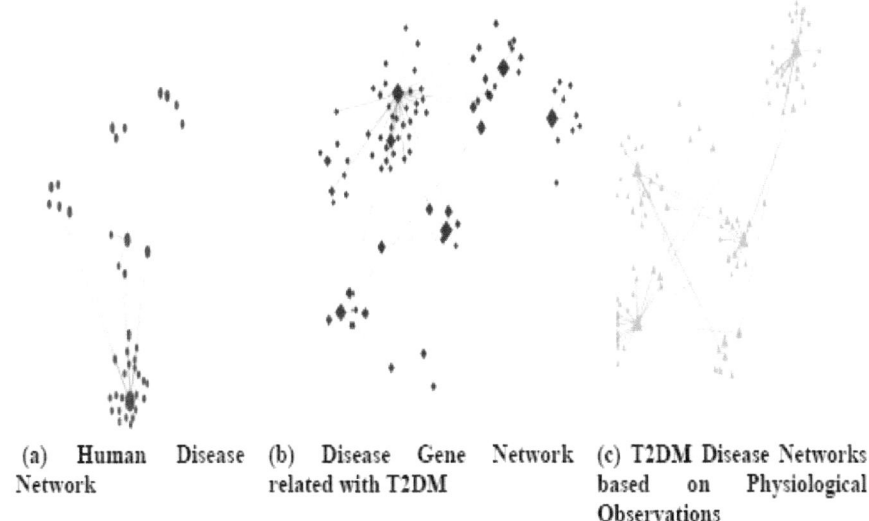

(a) Human Disease (b) Disease Gene Network (c) T2DM Disease Networks
Network   related with T2DM   based   on   Physiological
                                                        Observations

Fig. 4. Snapshot of single level T2DM networks [2]

Based on the multivariate and multidimensional association analysis (MMARCD) between genes and physiological data, we can construct the correlation network for disease, gene and physiological observations shown in Fig. 5, which is heterogeneous, hybrid and multilevel network. Fig. 5 is a small subset of T2DM-based disorder-disease gene and clinical trait associations, where circles correspond to the complex disease, rectangles correspond to physiological observations, and diamonds correspond to the disease genes. A link is placed between complex disease, clinical observations and genes that change together. The size of circles is proportional to the number of genes and observations participating in the corresponding disorder, and distance between the nodes is proportional to the correlation measurement. The correlation network will offer a platform to explore phenotype and disease gene associations in a multidimensional graph theoretic framework, indicating the genetic origin of T2DM.

The correlation networks combined with the classification methods can learn the pattern from the two datasets in the categories of T2DM and non-T2DM. Using the learned patterns, new patients with genetic variation and physiological change data can be diagnosed accurately and efficiently into the two categories. In the prognosis analysis of T2DM, the system can learn the historical patterns to predict future patterns in the same patients and learn similar patterns from other diagnosed patients [2]. Combining the patients' historical patterns and similar patterns learned from previous patients, this system could predict the further development of T2DM for the patients in a more accurate and repeatable way.

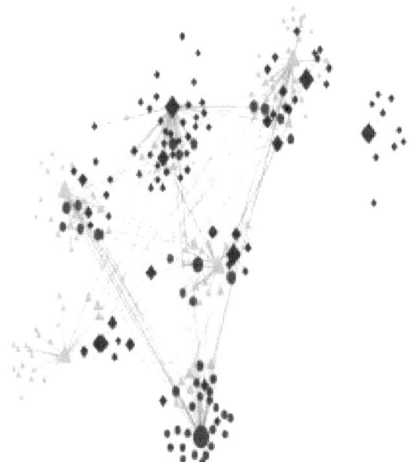

Fig. 5. Construction of the correlation network

5   Conclusion

In this paper, we propose a novel approach, Multivariate and Multidimensional Association Rule mining system based on Change Detection (MMARCD), to assist medical professionals to identify relationships between genetic variation, physiological change (e.g. in blood pressure or weight) and a disease or syndrome such as T2DM. Based upon MMARCD, a correlation network can be constructed to diagnose and prognose the development of human diseases.

For the future work, we would like to implement and optimise the association rules. We will also visualise the correlation disease network in a more effective and efficient way.

References

1. Botstein, D., Risch, N.: Discovering genotypes underlying human phenotypes: past successes for mendelian disease, future approaches for complex disease. Nature Genetics 33, 228–237 (2003), doi: 10.1038
2. He, J., Zhang, Y., Huang, G.: Multivariate association mining for genetics and physiological data related with T2DM. Health Information Science and Systems (October 2011) (accepted)
3. Christensen, K., Murray, J.: What genome-wide association studies can do for medicine. N Engl. J. Med. 356(11), 1169–1171 (2007)
4. Klein, R.: Complement factor H polymorphism in age-related macular degeneration. Science 308, 385–389 (2005), PMID, 15761122
5. Johnson, A., O'Donnell, C.: An open access database of genome-wide association results. BMC Medical Genetics 10(6) (2009)

6. CGEMS Data Access, Cancer Genetic Markers of Susceptibility, National Cancer Institute, U.S.A., http://cgems.cancer.gov/
7. National Human Genome Research Institute, National Institutes of Health, http://www.genome.gov/
8. Diabetes Genetics Initiative, http://www.braod.mit.edu/diabetes
9. Ku, C.: The pursuit of GWA studies: where are we now? Journal of Human Genetics 55(4), 195–206 (2010)
10. Sladek, R., Rocheleau, G., Rung, J., et al.: A GWAS identifies novel risk loci for type 2 diabetes. Nature 445(7130), 881–885 (2007)
11. Welcome Trust Case Control Consortium, Genome-wide association study of 14,000 cases of seven common diseases and 3,000 shared controls. Nature 447(7145), 661–678 (2007)
12. Kuok, C.M., Fu, A., Wong, M.H.: Shatin, Mining fuzzy association rules in databases. ACM SIGMOD 27(1) (1998)
13. Georgii, E., et al.: Analyzing microarray data using quantitative association rules. Bioinformatics 21(2), ii123–ii129
14. Agrawal, R., Srikant, R.: Fast algorithm for mining association rules in large databases. In: VLDB 1994, Santiago, Chile, pp. 487–499 (1994)
15. Pei, J., Han, J., Mao, R.: CLOSET: An efficient algorithm for mining frequent closed itemsets. In: Proc. 2000 ACM-SIGMOD Int. Workshop Data Mining and Knowledge Discovery (DMKD 2000), Dallas, TX, pp. 11–20 (May 2000)
16. Grahne, G., Zhu, J.: Efficiently using prefix-trees in mining frequent itemsets. In: Proc. ICDM 2003 Int. Workshop on Frequent Itemset Mining Implementations (FIMI 2003), Melbourne, FL (November 2003)
17. Zaki, M., Hsiao, C.: CHARM: An efficient algorithm for closed itemset mining. In: Proc. 2002 SIAM Int. Conf. Data Mining (SDM 2002), Arlington, VA, pp. 457–473 (April 2002)
18. Burdick, D., Calimlin, M., Gehrke, J.: MAFIA: A maximal frequent itemset algorithm for transactional databases. In: Proc. 2001 Int. Conf. Data Engineering (ICDE 2001), Heidelberg, Germany, pp. 443–452 (April 2001)
19. Ying, et al.: Predicting source code changes by mining revision history. IEEE Trans. Software Engineering 30, 574–586 (2004)
20. Zimmermann, et al.: Mining version histories to guide software changes. IEEE Trans. Software Eng. 31(6), 429–445 (2005)
21. Wu, et al.: Re-examination of interestingness measures in pattern mining: a unified framework. Data Min. Knowl. Discov. 21(3), 371–397 (2010)
22. Goh, K., Cusick, M., Valle, D., et al.: The human disease network. Proc. Natl. Acad. Sci., USA 104, 8685–8690 (2007)
23. Jimenez-Sanchez, G., Childs, B., Valle, D.: Human Disease Genes. Nature 409, 853–855
24. Childs, B., Valle, D.: Genetics, biology and disease. Annu. Rev. Genomics Hum. Genet. (1), 1–19 (2000)
25. Qiao, Z., He, J., Zhang, Y.: Multiple Time Series Anomaly Detection Based on Compression and Correlation Analysis: Algorithm and Medical Surveillance Case Study. In: 13th Asia Pacific Web Conference, Kunming, China (April 2012) (under review)
26. He, J., et al.: Cluster Analysis and Optimization in Color-Based Clustering for Image Abstract. In: ICDM Workshops 2007, pp. 213–218 (2007)
27. Huang, G., Ding, Z., He, J.: Automatic Generation of Traditional Style Painting by Using Density-Based Color Clustering. In: ICDM Workshops 2007, pp. 41–44 (2007)

28. MicroArray Gene Expression Markup Language Links,
    http://www.mged.org/Workgroups/MAGE/MAGEdescription2.pdf
29. Zhang, Y., Pang, C., He, J.: On multidimensional wavelet synopses for maximum error bounds. In: MCDM 2009, Chengdu, China (2009)
30. Huang, G., He, J., Ding, Z.: Wireless Video-Based Sensor Networks for Surveillance of Residential Districts. In: Zhang, Y., Yu, G., Bertino, E., Xu, G. (eds.) APWeb 2008. LNCS, vol. 4976, pp. 154–165. Springer, Heidelberg (2008)
31. Huang, G., He, J., Ding, Z.: Inter-frame change directing online clustering of multiple moving objects for video-based sensor networks. In: Web Intelligence/IAT Workshops 2008, pp. 442–446 (2008)
32. Han, J., Kamber, M.: Data Mining: Concepts and Techniques, 2nd edn. (2006)

Analysis of Nursery School Observations for Understanding Children's Behavior

Jien Kato and Yu Wang

Dept. of Systems and Social Informatics
Graduate School of Information Science, Nagoya University
Nagoya, Japan
jien@is.nagoya-u.ac.jp, ywang@nagoya-u.jp

Abstract. This paper introduces an on-going project with the goal of measuring and analyzing children's behavior automatically. Some key technologies, including methodologies for acquiring data, tracking a target across different cameras over time, activity recognition, interaction analysis, and behavior summarization for a target child are presented. Some encouraging results from a real system we developed in a nursery school environment are also described. As these technologies enable the content-based retrieval, comparison, and summarization of large-scale observational data, they are applicable to various purposes, such as the assessment of children's development, healthcare and diagnosis.

Keywords: activity recognition, interaction analysis, video summa-rization, behavior quantization, distance metric learning.

1   Introduction

The measurement and analysis of children's behavior, especially of those behaviors related to social and communication skills, are important for assessing children's development. For example, as remarked by specialists, children with Autism Spectrum Disorder (ASD) exhibit significant deficits in social interaction and communication [1]. The early recognition of risk for ASD may enable the at-risk children to benefit from therapy, which might effectively help to reduce the tremendous morbidity associated with this disorder.

To assess children's development in an objective way, it would be extremely helpful if the behavioral data of children could be measured in a natural environment across populations. In addition, it is also important to obtain long-term observational data of children's behavior as trend information over time is critical for the accurate assessment of children's developmental progress. On the other hand, it is not feasible to accumulate such a large quantity of data (for months or years) and to further extract valuable information from it manually.

From this viewpoint, we are conducting a project called MIMAMORI[1], which aims to study children's behavior by developing a system to automatically record and analyze the daily life of children in a nursery school environment. This paper presents

---

[1] A Japanese word means "watching affectionately".

J. He et al. (Eds.): HIS 2012, LNCS 7231, pp. 143–151, 2012.
© Springer-Verlag Berlin Heidelberg 2012

some key techniques that we have developed, including methodologies for acquiring data, tracking a target across cameras, recognizing activity, analyzing interactions and summarizing behavior for a specific target child [2], [3].

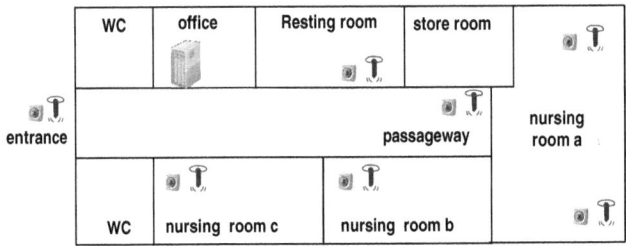

Fig. 1. Hardware configuration for data sensing

2   Core Technological Problems

In the MIMAMORI project, we record children's daily lives by the use of video, audio and temporal-spatial tags of moving targets. However, to protect privacy, we have not yet utilized the audio portion. As described above, our goal is to obtain an automated measurement and analysis of children's behavior using large-scale observational data. To achieve this goal, we face the following technological problems:

- Tracking a target child across multiple cameras
- Recognizing a target child's activities,
- Analyzing a target child's interactions with people.

The remaining paper is organized as follows: Section 3 shows our system setting; Section 4 describes the method for tracking a target child across multiple cameras over time; Section 5 presents activity recognition and interaction analysis; experimental results are shown in Section 6.

3   System Setting

We set up a data-sensing system in the nursery school within Nagoya University campus, which consists of seven cameras, each integrated with a RFID (Radio

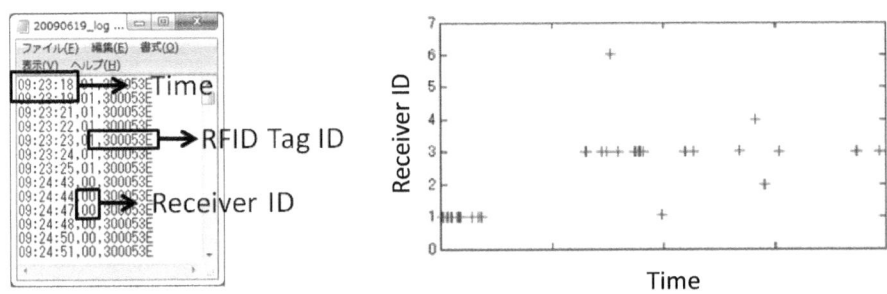

Fig. 2. Sample format of a RFID log (left) and visualization of some records (right). As receivers are set physically close to each other, there is some noise within the logs.

Frequency Identification) receiver. All of the seven camera-receiver pairs are installed in places where the children regularly appear: one in the entrance, four in the nursing rooms, one in the resting room and one in the passageway, as shown in Fig.1. Data recording from these seven locations occurs ten hours a day throughout the year.

Each camera is placed adjacent to an RFID receiver, which catches the signals sent by nearby RFID tags. Upon entering the nursery school each morning, every child is given an RFID tag to keep in his/her pocket. Subsequently, the tags will continuously send out the holder's ID, and the nearby receivers can capture the IDs and write them into a log file. This log information will later be used to effectively pick out videos that are expected to contain a specific child (called target-specific videos).

4   Tracking a Target Child in the Captured Data

To accumulate information about any target, we must be able to track moving people not only across multiple cameras, but on the recorded video stream taken by a single came. Here, we only discuss the former issue, as to the latter, we apply traditional visual tracking techniques.

The RFID log file consists of a number of records, as shown in Fig. 2 (left). Although such a record could be considered to be evidence that a specific child appears on the video stream captured by the camera adjacent to the RFID receiver, in practice, the signals are sometimes missed by all receivers and are sometimes captured by the wrong receiver because of interference (Fig. 2, right). To fix this problem and obtain the reliable extraction of target-specific videos, we introduce a weighted voting criterion.

We use one minute as a unit time interval that corresponds to n records in the log file, each with a receiver ID (ID_i). We then introduce a weight operator a_i for receiver ID_i that reflects the sensitivity of this receiver, particularly in the boundary areas where the signals might be sensed by other receivers. The weight a_i can be automatically estimated with the ground truth data or through manual assignment. We then obtain the votes v_i for each receiver within unit time T and select the receiver C as the camera according to

$$C = \arg\max_i a_i v_i (i \in \{1, \cdots, 7\}).$$

We repeat this procedure for all of the unit time intervals to obtain the target-specific videos that have high expectations of including the target.

5   Using the Template Analyzing a Target's Activities and Interactions with People

Given that we are able to follow a specified child over time, we want to measure behavioral variables by a computer vision-based approach that enables not only the characterization of, but ideally the quantification of, behavioral data automatically on a large scale. In the following, we describe how to recognize four types of regular activities in a nursery school and how to analyze the interactions between a target child and his/her peers during play time.

5.1   Activity Recognition

We define four types of regular chief activities in a day of a nursery school: eating, sleeping, playing and group activity. Because any activity lasts much longer than one minute, here we still use one minute as the unit time interval and divide the video into one minute segments before recognition.

We attack the activity recognition issue by first classifying every video segment into one of the chief activities through supervised classification and then by unsupervised clustering to discover individual activity clusters. Both the classification and the clustering are achieved with a learned Mahalanobis distance metric that appropriately measures the similarity between video segments.

1) Visual Features

For classification and clustering, we encode video segments into feature vectors with edge response, HOG distance, interframe subtraction and color histograms to cover a broad variety of activities (Fig. 3). The importance of these measurements will be encoded in the Mahalanobis distance metric. The features are as follows:

- *Edge response (f_e, 48-D), for describing the global appearance of a scene,*
- *Inter-frame subtraction (f_i, 48-D), for acquiring the global motion intensity between frames,*
- *HOG distance (f_h, 234-D), for capturing the local motion,*
- *Color histogram (f_c, 512-D), for characterizing the background of a scene.*

With the features computed for each frame as described above, we can acquire a 1684-D feature vector for a unit video segment by calculating the average and variance of these features:

$$(f_e^{\mu}, f_e^{\sigma}, f_i^{\mu}, f_i^{\sigma}, f_h^{\mu}, f_h^{\sigma}, f_c^{\mu}, f_c^{\sigma})^T$$

2) Distance Metric Learning

The objective of distance metric learning is to learn a Mahalanobis distance function,

$$Dist(f_n, f_m) = (f_n - f_m)^T M (f_n - f_m),$$

which measures the similarity of two feature vectors f_n and f_m. The state-of-the-art method for learning this M is known as a large margin nearest neighbor (LMNN) classification [4], in which, given the neighbor membership in a feature space, the M is obtained by minimizing the cost function,

$$L(M) = \sum_{i,j} w_i Dist_M(f_i, f_j) + C \sum_{i,j,k} w_i h\big(Dist_M(f_i, f_k) - Dist_M(f_i, f_j)\big),$$

Using an algorithm called semi-definitive programming (SDP). In the cost function, the first item penalizes the large distance between data point i and its target neighbors j (the neighbors that have the same label as point i), while the second item enforces point i to have a greater distance to imposter points k (the neighbors that have a different label with point i) than to the target neighbors j.

Because of the complicated situation present in this work, where the feature vector is a mixture of different kinds of features, and some dimensions of the vector might be very noisy for learning, we have proposed an extended LMNN method called Adapt LMNN to enhance the robustness of LMNN. The key idea of this extension is to introduce a binary feature mask into the cost function so that it becomes:

$$L(M) = \sum_{i,j} w_i Dist_M(\Phi \otimes f_i, \Phi \otimes f_j)$$
$$+ C \sum_{i,j,k} w_i h\big(Dist_M(\Phi \otimes f_i, \Phi \otimes f_k) - Dist_M(\Phi \otimes f_i, \Phi \otimes f_j)\big),$$

where $\otimes$ specifies an element-wise multiplication to remove effects stemming from some indiscriminative dimensions of the feature vector. The mask Φ can be obtained by learning its discriminability for all features.

3) Activity Classification and Clustering

With the learned distance metric, for a novel video segment, we find its k nearest neighbors in the training set and apply the majority rule to assign chief activity labels. Activity recognition is an open-ended problem, which means that we would like to identify as many different activities as possible; moreover, in the high-dimensional feature space (1648-D in our case), each class is actually too coarse to be addressed in the subsequent processing. We therefore further conduct clustering to discover individual activity clusters within each chief class by applying the agglomerative clustering method.

5.2 Interaction Analysis

The objective of the interaction analysis is to quantify how a target child interacts with his/her peers or teachers. Interaction analysis is a very deep research topic. At present, we are only able to give a quantitative description of how much a target child interacts with his/her surrounding persons by measuring the number of these persons over time.

To accomplish this, for every frame within the video segments that are classified as "playing", we extract the target-child-centered-image patch. We compute the HOG feature for each of these patches, and adapt a pre-trained binary classifier to determine if such a patch includes an interaction (according to the number of persons surrounding the target). The classification results for all of the frames are accumulated and are then used to compute the rate of the frames (w) that include the interaction. We give an estimation for the target child as 1) quiet if $w<30\%$; 2) normal if $30\leq w<70\%$; or 3) active if $w\geq70\%$. The thresholds are determined by experience.

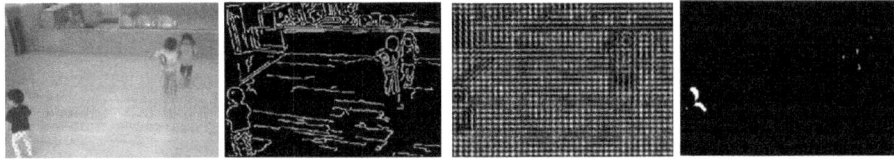

Fig. 3. Feature examples, from the left: input, edge, HOG and inter-frame subtraction

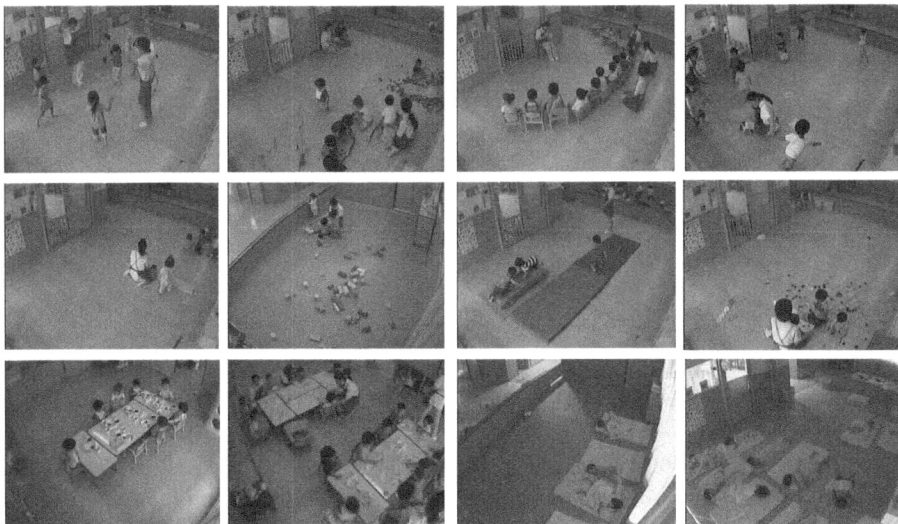

Fig. 4. Examples of clustering results, 1st row: group activity, 2nd row: playing, 3rd row left: eating, 3rd row right: sleeping

6   Experimental Results

We have implemented a system in a real nursery school environment to record the daily life of children and to analyze their activities and interactions by the proposed technologies. The performance of the system has been evaluated in different aspects that are summarized below.

Table 1. Results of Chief Activit Recognition

Test	Playing	Group Activity	Sleeping	Eating	Average
LMNN	80.5%	35.4%	82.5%	70.3%	71.3%
ALMNN	95.1%	78.8%	96.7%	89.7%	91.7%

Table 2. Activity Statistics for a Specific Child in a Single Day (m: minute)

Test	Group Activity	Eating	Playing	Sleeping	Total
Labeled Time	135 m	57 m	153 m	150 m	495 m
Estimated Time	142 m	53 m	161 m	139 m	495 m
Estimated Occupation	28.7%	10.7%	32.5%	28.1%	100%
Estimation Error	5.19%	7.02%	5.23%	7.33%	6.19%

Table 3. Results of Questionnaire

Question	A is better	Nearly identical	B is better
Q1	3	11	1
Q2	2	12	1

6.1   Activity Recognition

The objective of chief activity recognition is to predict a chief class label for each video segment. To evaluate our proposed activity recognition method, we prepared a manually labeled data set that consists of 3486 video segments taken from two-day videos: 471 for eating, 734 for sleeping, 1639 for playing, and 642 for group activity. We also prepared a test data set that includes 1162 video segments taken from videos on other days: 155 for eating, 246 for sleeping, 549 for playing, and 212 for group activity.

From the training data, we learned a Mahanalobis distance metric with our Adaptive LMNN. In the test step, we found the five nearest neighbors of each test video segment in the training data set with the learned distance metric and assigned the segment a class label by adapting the majority rule. The accuracy for activity recognition is shown in Table 1. For comparison, we also implemented the original LMNN using the same testing and training data, and we summarize the results in this same table. Comparing our method to the original LMNN, our proposed method achieved much better recognition accuracy.

After dividing all of the video segments into four chief activity groups, we further conducted clustering using the same distance metric. This clustering results in multiple clusters within each chief class. We pick out the centroid of large clusters and display their middle frames in Fig. 4. The misclassification that occurs in the chief activity recognition step does not have a large effect on the clustering results.

6.2   Interaction Analysis

The accuracy of the interaction analysis is confirmed through a patch classification experiment. We manually labeled 296 child-centered image patches. Two thirds of them are used for training, and 1/3 of them are used for testing. In the experiment, the patches are resized to 60×60 pixels and are computed into a 900-D HOG feature vector. We trained a linear SVM from the training data, and we adapted it to classify the testing data. The precision is approximately 87%.

6.3   Summarization of Children's Behavior

1) Behavior Quantization

We selected one child as the target and automatically analyzed his activities for one day. The resulting statistics are summarized into a daily report, shown in Table 2. In this experiment, to evaluate the accuracy of our system, we also manually classified the test data. From Table 2, we can see that the proposed system can conduct activity recognition very well: the report indicates that this child has spent 28.7%, 10.7%, 32.5%, and 28.1% of his time in a single day in group activity, eating, playing and sleeping, respectively, with an estimation error rate near 6%.

2) Video Digest Generation

We invited another child to spend a whole day with an RFID tag in his pocket. After picking out his target-specific video, we applied our proposed methods to identify chief activity labels and cluster labels within the groups for individual video segments. We also clipped out a patch video that concentrated on the target child and applied our proposed method to analyze his interactions with his peers during playing and group activity time.

We generated a one-day video digest by choosing video segments that accurately reflect the child's situation and connecting them temporally. The video segments are chosen under the following criteria:

- to include as many segments as possible that belong to different chief classes and clusters,
- to include as many segments as possible where the target child interacts with his/her peers,
- to make the digest easy for understanding the daily life of the target child.

To evaluate the quality of the generated digest, we also produced a digest manually using the same raw data under the same criteria for digest organization. We invited a group of 15 parents and nursery school teachers to participate in our questionnaire survey. They are asked to watch two unmarked digest videos and answer the following questions:

Q1.   Which video is better?

Q2.   Which video better describes the child's daily life?

The answers are summarized in Table 3. From the results, we can see that most people think that video B (automatically generated) is almost identical to video A (manually generated). That is to say, using our proposed activity recognition method, it is possible to summarize children's behavior automatically.

7   Conclusion

We have introduced our on-going project MIMAMORI, which aims to automatically measure and analyze children's behavior. Some key technologies, including those for acquiring data, tracking a target across cameras over time, identifying individuals, recognizing activities, analyzing interactions, and summarizing behavior for a specific child, are presented. Experimental results from a real system installed in a nursery school are very encouraging. As these technologies enable the content-based retrieval, comparison, and summarization of large-scale observational data, they are applicable to various purposes, such as healthcare and diagnosis for children or the elderly. In future works, it will be necessary to analyze people's activities and interactions in further detail.

References

1. Charman, T., Baird, G.: Practitioner Review: Diagnosis of Autism Spectrum Disorder in 2- and 3-year-old Children. Journal of Child Psychology and Psychiatry 43(3), 289–305 (2002)
2. Ishikawa, T., Wang, Y., Kato, J.: Daily Digest Generation of Kindergartner from Surveillance Video. IEEJ Transactions on Electronics, Information and Systems 131(2), 385–392 (2011) (in Japanese)
3. Kato, J., Ishikawa, T., Wang, Y., Ishii, K.: Video Digest Generation with Multisensor for Nursery School Kids. ICIC Express Letters 5(6), 1921–1927 (2011)
4. Weinberger, K.Q., Saul, K.: Distance Metric Learning for Large Margin Nearest Neighbour Classification. Journal of Machine Learning Research 10, 207–244 (2009)

Epidemic Outbreak and Spread Detection System Based on Twitter Data

Xiang Ji[1], Soon Ae Chun[2], and James Geller[1]

[1] New Jersey Institute of Technology, Newark, NJ, USA
{xj25,geller}@njit.edu
[2] CUNY College of Staten Island, Staten Island, NY, USA
{soon.chun}@csi.cuny.edu

Abstract. Social Network systems, such as Twitter, can serve as important data sources to provide collective intelligence and awareness of health problems in real time. The challenges of utilizing social media data include that the volume of data is large but distributed and of a highly unstructured form. Appropriate data gathering, scrubbing and aggregating efforts for these data are required to transform them for meaningful use. In this paper, we discuss such a social media data ETL (Extract-Transform-Load) method, to provide a user-friendly, dynamic method for visualizing outbreaks and the spread of developing epidemics in space and time. We have developed the Epidemics Outbreak and Spread Detection System (EOSDS) as a prototype that makes use of the rich information retrievable in real time from Twitter. EOSDS provides three different visualization methods of spreading epidemics, static map, distribution map, and filter map, to investigate public health threats in the space and time dimensions. The results of these visualizations in our experiments correlate well with relevant CDC official reports, a gold standard used by health informatics scientists. In our experiments, the EOSDS also detected an unusual situation not shown in the CDC reports, but confirmed by online news media.

Keywords: Social Network, Twitter, Epidemics Detection, Health Information Visualization, Epidemics Distribution, Epidemics Spread.

1 Introduction

Monitoring threats to public health is important for the healthcare community. The Web has created unprecedented resources for tracking such threats. A previous approach by Ginsberg to this problem relied exclusively on search engines, in which users could input queries in reference to issues they were most concerned about [1]. In their thread of research, such queries were recorded by a search engine provider, leading to the realization that an aggregation of large numbers of queries might show patterns that are useful for the early detection of disease outbreaks.

Ginsberg used Google's search query data (mostly keywords and phrases) to generate an early detection system, which could report outbreaks of influenza roughly two weeks prior to the official report of influenza. The official report is based on the

J. He et al. (Eds.): HIS 2012, LNCS 7231, pp. 152–163, 2012.

number of patient visits to local hospitals and published by the Centers for Disease Control and Prevention (CDC).

However, the research on the detection of epidemics based on search queries is limited by two factors: First, user input query terms are regarded by search engine corporations as their core assets and are not available to outside researchers. Second, user locations are not explicitly recorded. As the users enter keywords into the search engine, the queries and IP addresses are recorded. However, the IP addresses, which can be converted to actual user locations, are not easily accessible to outsiders; thus, it is difficult to develop applications which use the actual geographic locations of users.

Twitter, a micro-blog service provider, is showing great potential for overcoming the limitations stated above. There are more than 230 million tweets posted by Twitter users per day [2]. What appears to be more important for researchers, however, is that most of the tweets are public. Moreover, the Twitter streaming API [3] enables researchers to retrieve everything contained in a tweet, including the people mentioned, the URLs, and the topic tag added by Twitter users. The users' geographic information is available in the form of physical addresses specified in user profiles.

Aramaki et al. used different machine learning models to classify influenza-related tweets into two categories [4]. With a window size of 6, the Support Vector Machine method achieved an F-measure of 0.756 in distinguishing relevant tweets, such as "I caught a flu, I was burning up," from tweets, such as "influenza is now raging through Japan," that are irrelevant to the location of the tweeter.

By analyzing a random sample of 500 Twitter users and their geographic locations, we found that 30% are left blank, 10% are spam addresses, like "in the universe" or "right behind you." The other 60% are valid addresses; however, they are distributed over different levels of granularity. For example, 78.3% of the valid addresses are "places," such as "NYC"; 12.5% are "states"; and 7.5% are "countries." Considering the above complexity of geographic names, if they are not properly processed, the subsequent estimation based on the addresses could easily lead to imprecise results. For example, in the data recorded on October 5th, 2011 by the influenza system "INFLUkun" [4], out of the 1,931 tweets, there were a total of 891 tweets whose locations were unrecognized. Unless the data with uncertain locations are interpreted correctly, there is the potential that the system could return a misleading result.

To address this issue, our Epidemics Outbreak and Spread Detection System (EOSDS) integrates a module to preprocess noisy geographic names. It applies a frequency-based delete list to identify and filter out non-informative geographic information, and it has the ability to detect different granularity levels of geographic names. To enhance the visual analytics of the disease outbreak detection, EOSDS provides three mapping techniques for tweets. A static map displays tweet instances about a relevant disease, while a distribution map displays numbers of tweets from different states in the US. A third display mode, the filter map, includes combined geospatial, temporal and user influence filters that provide a dynamic interface for a user to track tweet patterns for monitoring epidemic activity.

The rest of the paper is organized as follows. In Section 2, we introduce the EOSDS system. Section 3 is a detailed description of EOSDS and the visualization methods used. In Section 4, the visualization results are illustrated, interpreted, and discussed. Section 5 contains conclusions and suggests future research.

2   Overview of the EOSDS System

To better display the geographic locations of outbreaks and the spread of epidemics at multiple levels, we have developed the Epidemics Outbreak and Spread Detection System (EOSDS). Its architecture is shown in Figure 1. We used Twitter search and streaming APIs and phirehose libraries provided by 140dev [5], to build the data collector. It gathers the real-time tweets containing certain specified health-related keywords (e.g. listeria), along with associated user profile information for subsequent analysis into our local relational database. As stated above, tweets are noisy in terms of geographic locations. To filter out the roughly 40% of tweets which contain meaningless location terms, we manually selected a sample with meaningless locations and fed these terms into a text mining tool called Automap [6] to function as a "filter" to throw out meaningless locations from the remaining tweets.

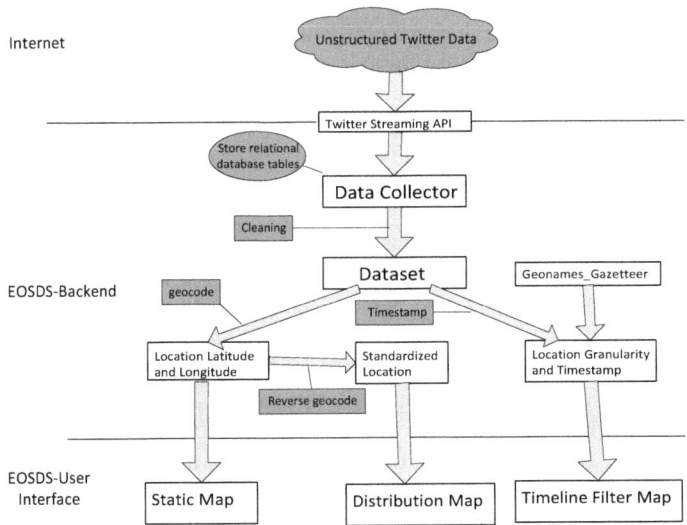

Fig. 1. Architecture of Epidemics Outbreak and Spread Detection System (EOSDS)

To serve different needs of epidemics detection, three kinds of map visualizations are generated. The *static map* is used to show the tweets based on "single" users' locations. In the distribution map, absolute and relative frequencies of the distribution are displayed. The relative frequency is the absolute frequency divided by the population of each state. The distribution map enables the detection of which states house most Twitter users tweeting about an epidemic. The filter map gives users the flexibility to monitor the spread of epidemics based on time series and users' influence with a (minimum, maximum) range of followers to only display Twitter users in this range. Monitoring population behavior at different levels of granularity is also possible in filter map mode, as the lower level granularities such as "place" will often indicate more precise estimates of actual locations than higher level granularities such as "country."

3   Methods of Epidemics Outbreak and Spread Detection System

3.1   Data Collection and Preprocessing

The overall processing can be described as ETL (Extract-Transform-Load) approach. We have been monitoring five popular epidemics: "tuberculosis," "listeria," "influenza." "swine flu," and "measles." Whenever a Twitter user posts a tweet containing one of the above disease names, that tweet and its related information is automatically preprocessed and recorded by EOSDS in the form of a relational database. The core PHP code for collecting epidemics related real-time tweets from the Twitter Streaming API is illustrated in Figure 2.

```
class Consumer extends Phirehose

{

        public function enqueueStatus($status) {

                $tweet_object = json_decode($status);

                ......

        }

}

$stream=new Consumer (STREAM_ACCOUNT,

STREAM_PASSWORD, Phirehose::METHOD_FILTER);

$stream->db_connect();

$stream->setTrack(array('health'));

$stream->consume();
```

Fig. 2. PHP code for retrieving real-time epidemics related tweets

In Figure 2, the PHP code creates a class "Consumer;" "health" is the keyword we want to watch in this example. The call to consume() will activate enqueueStatus() to automatically collect tweets and store them into the local MySQL database tables. The database structure of EOSDS is shown in Figure 3.

3.1.1   Location Preprocessing

We filter the locations recorded in the Twitter profiles of "tweeters" by using location stop words. We manually selected 100 meaningless locations, such as "in the universe" and "wherever you are." We then fed these locations to the concept list generator module in Automap [8]. Automap is a text mining and network text analysis tool. Its concept list functionality takes a text file as input, and outputs each concept with its number of occurrences (frequency) in the input file.

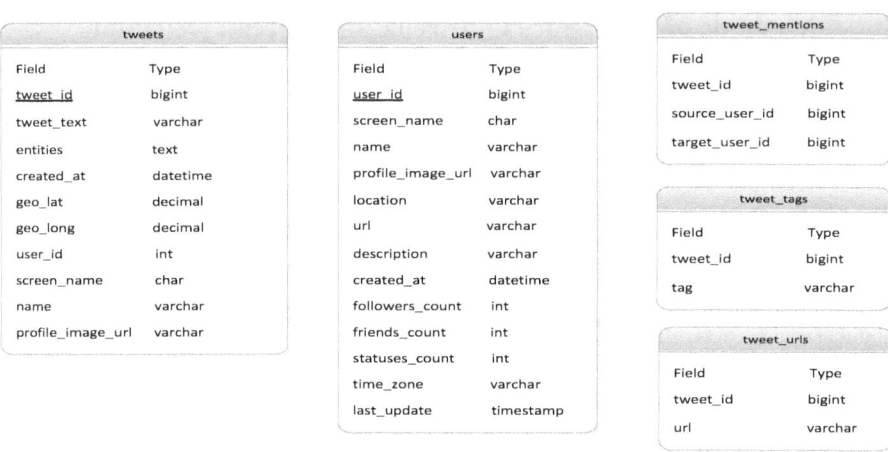

Fig. 3. EOSDS relational database tables for storing tweet information

We generated a list of "single-grams" (concepts which contain exactly one word) in descending order of term frequency that most likely occur in meaningless locations. Table 1 shows the top five single-grams. The list is adopted by EOSDS as the delete list. The delete list was applied to a test dataset, which contained 1000 records that were posted by Twitter users. The results are shown in Table 2. Of these 1000, 354 locations were categorized as spam by EOSDS. According to a manual check, 362 records were actually spam locations. Thus, EOSDS achieved a precision of 97.1%, and a recall of 95.8% in identifying meaningless locations.

3.2 Static Map

The static map display mode provides a direct way to display locations of all tweet instances. After the preprocessing, only records containing valid geographic information are left. Before mapping the geographic information to the actual map, EOSDS geocodes the geographic information into (latitude, longitude) coordinates that can be processed by the system. EOSDS' geocoding is done by the Google Map API [7]. Every location is passed to the geocoding server, and the returned latitude and longitude are mapped by EOSDS to show the estimated location of each tweet.

Table 1. Top five single-grams in meaningless locations

Concept	Frequency	Relative Frequency	Gram Type
the	19	1.00	single
In	17	0.89	single
in	13	0.68	single
The	8	0.42	single
you	8	0.42	single

Table 2. Result of identifying spam address. Detect+ means the locations that are identified as spam addesses. S+ means the locations that are in fact spam addresses.

	S– (not spam)	S+ (spam)	Total
Detect+	7	347	354
Detect–	631	15	646
Total	638	362	1000

We assume that the location information specified in a user profile is the location where the user actually posted the tweet, probably the place where s/he lives or works. In the case of tweets posted by mobile devices like smart phones, we skip the step of geocoding and use the mobile devices' location at the time of tweeting (this location is also recorded in the EOSDS database) as the user's actual location.

The static map provides a straight forward way to monitor the tweet users' concerns about an epidemic. However, we desire to gain "the big picture" in terms of the geographic distribution of disease-related tweets and the spread of the public's concerns about epidemics. The above two goals are achieved by the distribution map and filter map as will be shown below.

3.3   Distribution Map and Two Step Coding

The idea of building a distribution map is based on a problem with the static map. In the static map, we have many markers which represent individual users who are posting tweets. We can visually recognize wherever there is an unusual cluster of "markers," which should be investigated by public health officials. In the static map, it is not always easy to judge whether a particular area is unusual, because different people may have different criteria for tweeting. Another limitation with the static map is that in some states such as California, there are more tweets because there are more people than in other states. But is there always an epidemic in these areas? Thus, the display needs to be corrected according to the population distribution.

The above problems are addressed by the distribution map. To build the distribution map, we need to know what state a particular tweet comes from. But the users' profile locations, even after the data cleaning introduced in Section 3.1, lie at different levels of granularity. The granularity of locations creates a difficulty to identify what state or city a tweet comes from. EOSDS solves this problem by a method we call "two-step coding." The different levels of granularity are shown in Table 3.

Table 3. Different levels of granularity

Granularity	Example
Place	Newark, New Jersey
State	Colorado
Country	Netherlands
World	heaven

We use the method of two-step coding as follows. First we geocode all the locations into latitudes and longitudes, then we reversely geocode the obtained latitudes and longitudes into standardized addresses. For example, at the place level, some user-specified locations are "Rochester," "Rochester, USA," "NYC." At the state level, some locations are "NY," or "New York." In the geocoding step, "Rochester" and "Rochester, USA" are translated into latitudes and longitudes indicating the downtown area of the city of Rochester in the state of New York. "NYC," "NY," and "New York" are geocoded into latitude and longitude pointing to downtown Manhattan (even if the user is located in Brooklyn). We then apply reverse geocoding, converting latitude and longitude into physical addresses. We retrieve these addresses in the format "county, state, country" or "state, country." Thus, after two-step coding, "Rochester" and "Rochester, USA" become identical, standardized addresses: "Monroe, New York, USA." "NYC," "NY," and "New York" become standardized into "New York, USA." With standardized addresses, our system knows how many tweets (absolute frequency) are from each state. The whole process is illustrated in the Figure 4.

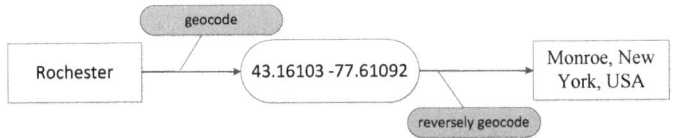

Fig. 4. The process of two step coding

Besides absolute frequency, the relative frequency of each state is calculated as the absolute frequency of each state divided by the population of the state (normalized by a factor of 1,000,000). Thus, sparsely populated states gain a larger weight than densely populated states. This method makes the epidemics trend easier to monitor.

3.4   Filter Map

The filter map provides users with a dynamic interface to monitor and analyze dynamic trends derivable from health-related tweets. Three filters are incorporated into the filter map: granularity filter, influence filter and timeline filter.

3.4.1   Granularity Filter

Different levels of location granularity represent different precision levels. For example, "Newark, NJ" is more precise than "New Jersey." "New Jersey" is more precise than "United States." To match a certain location with a level of granularity, we make use of a gazetteer. A gazetteer is a geographical dictionary or directory, an important source of data about places and place names, used in conjunction with maps [8]. To label locations with the correct level of granularity, we utilized the "National Places Gazetteer" [9] issued by the U.S. Census Bureau as the standard resource.

The "National Places Gazetteer" contains more than 29,000 US places, including cities, towns, boroughs, and Census-designated places (CDP). These names represent the lowest level of granularity. Names of the 50 states and names of 245 countries worldwide are also used together with the National Places Gazetteer. Each location was checked against this extended gazetteer. There are cases of multiple records in the gazetteer matching a single location in the dataset, but we found that those multiple matching records almost always are at a single level of granularity. For example, there are a few locations in the US called "London," but all belong to a single granularity level: place. It is very rare that a name is shared by two levels of granularity, which means that we can achieve a high precision in matching locations with levels of granularity. Filtering with different levels of geographic locations allows making maximal use of the information available. If EOSDS users choose a map only showing the place-level locations, the displayed map positions provide a more accurate perspective for investigating the locations of the epidemic.

3.4.2   Influence Filter

Not every tweeter has the same impact on his environment. A range of follower counts may be set by an EOSDS user to display only those Twitter users with a number of followers greater than the minimum and smaller than the maximum. This functionality is helpful to find how the "influencers" are distributed over the map. The effect of applying the influence filter is illustrated in Figure 5. It enables the users to concentrate only on the tweets that are highly influential. By tracking the distribution of influential tweets, we can estimate where the "seed tweet" originated, and how these influential tweets affect the spread of public concern about a certain epidemic.

3.4.3   Timeline Filter

Besides the space dimension, considering that every tweet has a timestamp, tweets can also provide us with an additional perspective to gain insights into the temporal distribution and development of an epidemic. The timeline filter was built with SIMILE [10]. By moving the time forward and backward, EOSDS users can easily find a particular time frame to recognize where and when a sudden increase of tweets occurs, and how this fits into the bigger picture of the epidemic.

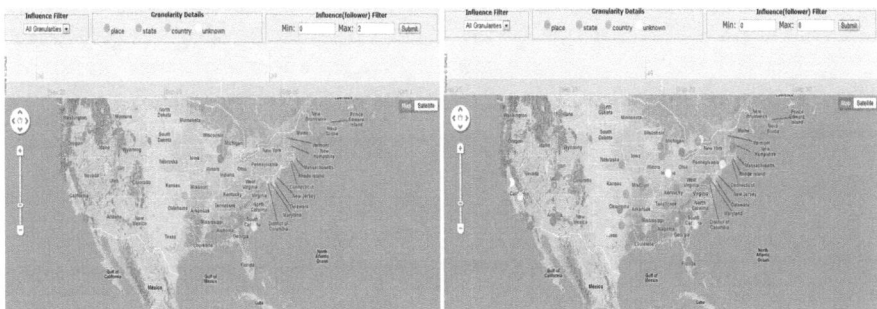

Fig. 5. The left figure shows the tweet users with influence range between 0 and 2. The right figure shows the tweet users with influence range between 0 and 8.

4   Visualization Results and Discussion

The test dataset was collected by EOSDS by specifying the keyword "listeria," and the monitoring period from "09-26-2011" to "09-28-2011," which is during a severe outbreak of listeria in North America. There are 2605 tweets in total, of which 920 tweets were removed by EOSDS data cleaning functionality. The result as a static map visualization is shown in Figure 6.

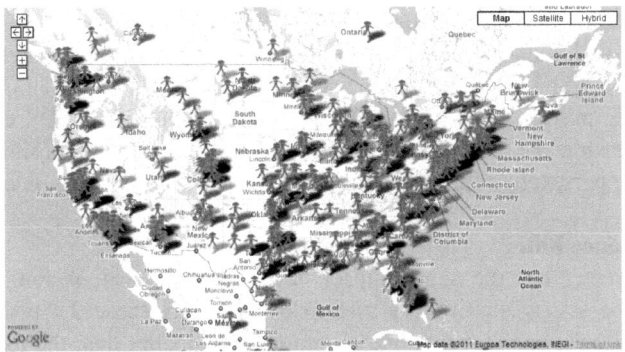

Fig. 6. Static map visualization result

In the visualization, EOSDS users can detect a few states with big clusters of Twitter users tweeting about "listeria." These states include California, Washington, Colorado, Texas, Arizona, Florida, Maryland, and New York. According to the CDC's report, as of 11am EDT on September 29, 2011, a total of 84 persons were infected with listeria. The states with the largest numbers of infected persons were identified as follows: Colorado (17), Texas (14), New Mexico (13), Oklahoma (11), Nebraska (6), Kansas (5) [11]. Therefore the static map showed good correlation with CDC reports. The distribution map's result is shown in Figure 8 and can be compared with the CDC's report on the listeria distribution, which was published three days later, as shown in Figure 7. The results also correlate well with the CDC report. Colorado, Texas, Kansas and Wyoming have the most Twitter users showing concerns about "listeria" in their tweets.

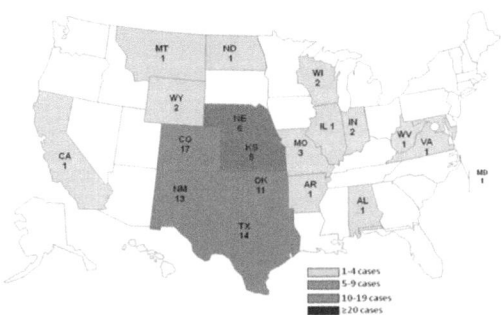

Fig. 7. Distribution map published by CDC on September 30th, 2011

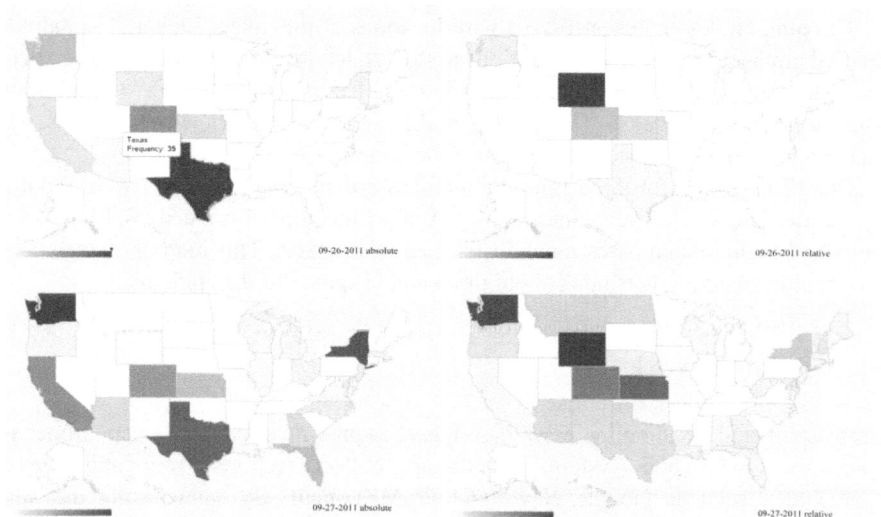

Fig. 8. The top shows absolute (left) and relative (right) frequency maps of 09-26-2011. The bottom shows absolute (left) and relative (right) frequency maps of 09-27-2011.

In the EOSDS distribution map, Wyoming is an unusual state. Wyoming's frequency is relatively low in the official CDC report, but its relative frequency is the highest in the EOSDS distribution map. The reason is that on September 26th, a death was confirmed by the health department of Wyoming [12], but that death was not in the CDC report until October 6th [13]. This shows that EOSDS can be used as an effective early warning system.

The filter map has the power to track the spread of an epidemic on a time line. The display of the filter map is shown in Figure 9.

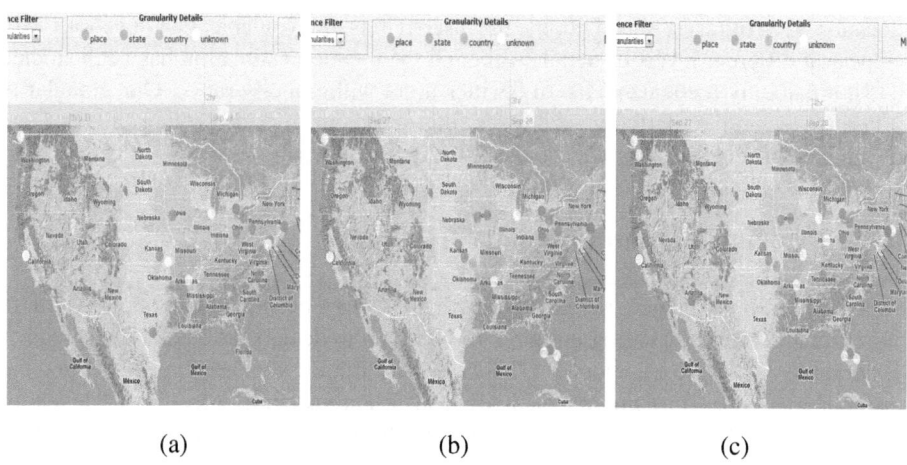

    (a)   (b)   (c)

Fig. 9. (a) timeline: 3:00 am; (b) timeline: 4:00 am; (c) timeline: 5:00 am

The pink circles represent tweets with locations at the "place" level. The salmon-colored circles are tweets with locations at the "state" level. The cyan circles indicate the tweets at the "country" level. The white circles are tweets at the "world" level. The "world level" means "anywhere in the world." In other words, colors with mnemonic names were chosen (e.g. Cyan for Country).

The visualization (at three time points) shows that the initial cases were reported by Twitter users all around the country. But as the time advanced, California and Maryland accumulated cases much faster than other states. This kind of change could give healthcare specialists hints about the possible spread of the epidemic.

5   Related Work

Brownstein et al. used online news-based data, to provide surveillance capabilities for epidemics [14]. Their system, Healthmap, collects reports from online news aggregators, such as Google News and ProMED-mail. By categorizing the news reports into epidemics-related items and unrelated reports, and filtering the epidemics-related documents into "breaking news," "warnings," and "old news," the system is able to trigger alerts based on the "breaking news."

With regards to location processing, a study by Cheng et al. determines users' positions when location information is absent. Their location estimator can place 51% of the Twitter users within 100 miles of their actual locations [15]. Their approach relies on detecting "local" words, which are of a high local specificity and a fast dispersion, such as "howdy" in Texas.

The EOSDS system described in this paper is different from the above research in terms of data sources and processing of locations. It is a current trend that social network sites, such as Twitter and PatientsLikeMe are surpassing search engines [1] and news portals [14] as main information sources. In terms of processing locations, it is important to provide levels of granularity, as presented in this paper. Because the location is arbitrarily specified by the users, it is unavoidable that locations will appear at different levels of detail. Although the location estimation has been studied [15], it can only recognize 51% of Twitter users within a city range. Our granularity filtering technique partially addresses this problem by identifying higher-level locations, thus makes maximal use of the available information.

6   Conclusions and Future Work

We have outlined the geographic aspects that have not been paid enough attention to by current research regarding utilizing Twitter data to detect and predict the spread of epidemics. We have developed EOSDS with modules to clean noisy geographic locations based on text mining methods, and to automatically identify the levels of granularity for different location specifications. Furthermore, EOSDS enables users to visualize the Twitter data from three different perspectives. The advantages and limitations of each map were discussed. In our experiments, all three maps displayed listeria patterns that correlated well with the CDC reports on the same topic. Also, the distribution map made it possible to discover an unusual listeria outbreak situation in Wyoming, which was not reported by the CDC until several days later.

The EOSDS system can be improved in the following aspects in the future: (i) Incorporate more names of other countries into the standard gazetteer; (ii) Analyze sentiments to quantify the "degree of worry" of each tweet; (iii) Introduce other parameters besides the number of followers, to improve the influence feature.

Acknowledgements. This work was supported in part by PSC-CUNY Research Grant 41 awarded to Soon Ae Chun.

References

1. Ginsberg, J., Mohebbi, M.H., Patel, R.S., Brammer, L., Smolinski, M.S., Brilliant, L.: Detecting influenza epidemics using search engine query data. Nature 457, 1012–1014 (2009)
2. Sipping from the fire hose: Making sense of a torrent of tweets. The Economist, p. 68 (2011)
3. Twitter developers documentation, https://dev.twitter.com/docs
4. Aramaki, E., Maskawa, S., Morita, M.: Twitter Catches The Flu: Detecting Influenza Epidemics using Twitter. In: Conference on Empirical Methods in Natural Language Processing, EMNLP 2011 (2011)
5. 140dev libraries, http://140dev.com/ (accessed on February 8, 2012)
6. Carley, K.M., Columbus, D., Bigrigg, M., Kunkel, F.: Automap user guide (2011)
7. Google Map API,
   http://code.google.com/apis/maps/documentation/geocoding/
8. Aurousseau, M.: On Lists of Words and Lists of Names. The Geographical Journal 105, 61–67 (1945)
9. National Places Gazetteer, http://www.census.gov/geo/www/
   gazetteer/files/Gaz_places_national.txt (accessed on February 8, 2012)
10. Mazzocchi, S., Garland, S., Lee, R.: SIMILE: practical metadata for the semantic web. O'Reilly (2005)
11. CDC Listeria report on September 30, http://www.cdc.gov/listeria/
    outbreaks/cantaloupes-jensen-farms/093011/index.html
12. Wyoming news report, http://www.health.wyo.gov/
    news.aspx?NewsID=498 (accessed on February 8, 2012)
13. CDC Listeria report on October 7, http://www.cdc.gov/listeria/
    outbreaks/cantaloupes-jensen-farms/100711/index.html
    (accessed on February 8, 2012)
14. Brownstein, J.S., Freifeld, C.C., Reis, B.Y., Mandl, K.D.: Surveillance Sans Frontières: Internet-Based Emerging Infectious Disease Intelligence and the HealthMap Project. PLoS Med. 5(7), e151 (2008), doi:10.1371/journal.pmed.0050151
15. Cheng, Z., Caverlee, J., Lee, K.: Proceedings of the 19th ACM International Conference on Information and Knowledge Management (CIKM 2010), Toronto, Canada, October 26-30 (2010)

A Lightweight Approach for Extracting Disease-Symptom Relation with MetaMap toward Automated Generation of Disease Knowledge Base

Takashi Okumura and Yuka Tateisi

National Institute of Public Health
2-3-6 Minami, Wako-shi, Saitama 351-0197, Japan
taka@niph.go.jp

Abstract. Diagnostic decision support systems necessitate disease knowledge base, and this part may occupy dominant portion in the total development cost of such systems. Accordingly, toward automated generation of disease knowledge base, we conducted a preliminary study for efficient extraction of symptomatic expressions, utilizing MetaMap, a tool for assigning UMLS (Unified Medical Language System) semantic tags onto phrases in a given medical literature text.

We first utilized several tags in the MetaMap output, related to symptoms and findings, for extraction of symptomatic terms. This straightforward approach resulted in Recall 82% and Precision 64%. Then, we applied a heuristics that exploits certain patterns of tag sequences that frequently appear in typical symptomatic expressions. This simple approach achieved 7% recall gain, without sacrificing precision.

Although the extracted information requires manual inspection, the study suggested that the simple approach can extract symptomatic expressions, at very low cost. Failure analysis of the output was also performed to further improve the performance.

1 Introduction

Disease Knowledge Base resides at the center of diagnostic decision support systems [14]. To suggest appropriate regimen for a patient, the support system examines the knowledge base for diseases that match the presented symptoms, and then, hooks the information associated with the suspected disease. Accordingly, the system utility depends on the quality and the coverage of the knowledge base.

It is, however, costly to compile a usable knowledge base. First of all, the number of diseases ever known counts up to six thousands [10], which boosts the maintenance cost of the knowledge base. Second, a disease may present a variety of symptoms with differing intensity and temporal variation, and thus, description of a disease is often provided in an unstructured free text format. Third, interpretation of the information requires medical background, which also expands the compilation cost of the knowledge base.

J. He et al. (Eds.): HIS 2012, LNCS 7231, pp. 164–172, 2012.

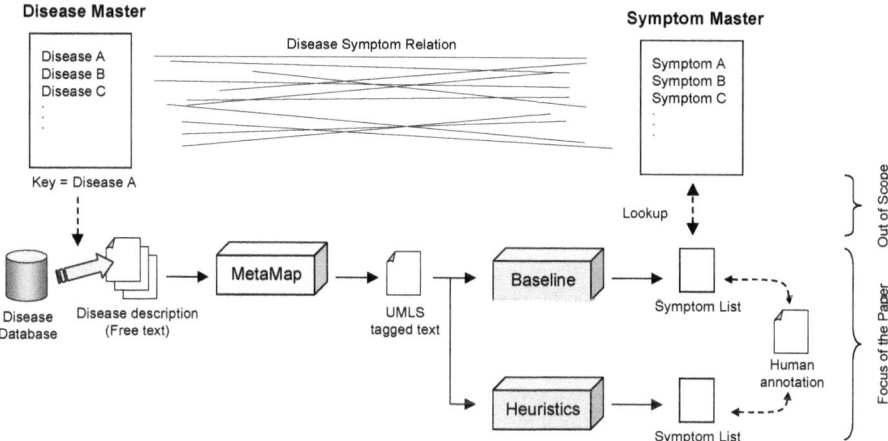

Fig. 1. Overview of the experiment

Accordingly, toward automated generation of disease knowledge base, we first need to extract symptomatic information for a certain disease, out of medical literature, written in natural language, at low cost. To this end, we utilized MetaMap [2,1,15], which maps phrases in medical text onto standardized UMLS (Unified Medical Language System) terminology [4], and applied simple rules to extract symptomatic expressions on the MetaMap output. Then, based on the analysis of the result, we devised simple heuristics, which exploits certain patterns that appear in symptomatic expressions.

The rest of the paper is organized as follows. First, we briefly describe the experimental setting and our heuristics. Results of the experiments are given in Section 3, which is followed by discussion in Section 4, with analysis of failure cases and future development. Section 5 summarizes related works, and we conclude the paper in Section 6.

2   Method

Overview. MetaMap is a program that converts a medical literature text into phrases, with terms mapped onto UMLS terminology, coupled with their semantic category. For example, a phrase, "retinal pigmentary changes" (appears in OMIM ID 118450) is automatically mapped to "retinal pigments" and "change", which are tagged as "Biologically Active Substance, Organic Chemical" and "Quantitative Concept" or "Functional Concept", respectively. In our approach, the tool was used to convert descriptions of diseases in free text format, into texts with UMLS tags (Figure 1). The generated output was then processed to extract symptomatic expressions by looking up a set of UMLS semantic categories (Baseline). We also introduced simple heuristic rules on the occurrence of

UMLS categories (Heuristics), as explained later in this section. The extraction results were evaluated by human annotation, used as gold standard.

Note that, the paper focuses on the extraction of simple disease-symptom relations, without statistics nor conditions. Further, we use the word, "symptom", as a generic term to denote any phenotype of the disease, such as clinical signs, laboratory results, pathological findings, etc. Lastly, the lookup operation against the symptom master, or the maintenance of the master data, is beyond the scope of the paper, as indicated in Figure 1.

Material. As the target text, we utilized OMIM [12], which is a widely used database of human genes and genetic disorders, by Johns Hopkins University. Each OMIM entry includes clinical features of the disorder, in free text, and the descriptions are used as input of our experiments. We used 20 free text descriptions of diseases on the database. Document IDs are 108450, 113450 118450, 123450, 140450, 176450, 181450, 200450, 203450, 214450, 218450, 233450 236450, 244450, 248450, 259450, 265450, 267450, 305450, and 311450, which were randomly selected.

Baseline rule. Based on MetaMap output of two texts (OMIM ID 118450 and 181450), we categorized the UMLS semantic tags into several groups, to extract symptomatic expressions. The most important group is the *SYMPTOM* group, because they are used for description of a symptom. For example, Acquired Abnormality, Anatomical Abnormality, Cell or Molecular Dysfunction, Congenital Abnormality, Disease or Syndrome, Finding, Injury or Poisoning, Mental or Behavioral Dysfunction, Neoplastic Process, Pathologic function, Sign or Symptom, and Virus, fell in the *SYMPTOM* group.

Heuristics. During the experiments, we found certain UMLS semantic tag sequences that frequently appear in failure cases. For example, a symptomatic expression, *yellowish eyes*, comprises a word for *qualifier* and a following *body part* noun. Based on the observation, we introduced additional groups, *QUALIFIER*, which refers to attributes or characteristics of something, such as *Organism Attribute, Qualitative Concept, Quantitative Concept* etc., and *BODYPART* for semantic tags related to body location, such as *Body Part Organ or Organ Component, Cell Component, Tissue,* etc. Similarly, we added *ACTION* (*Behavior, Daily or Recreational Activity, Individual Behavior* etc.) and *FUNCTION* (*Biologic Function, Functional Concept, Chemical Viewed Functionally* etc.) groups, for human activities and functions of organisms or substances, respectively.

The groups are defined as follows.

- **ACTION group:** tags related to human activities

  Behavior, Daily or Recreational Activity, Environmental Effect of Humans, Human-caused Phenomenon or Process, Individual Behavior, Social Behavior, Therapeutic or Preventive Procedure

- **BODYPART group:** tags related to anatomy

  Body Location or Region, Body Part Organ or Organ Component, Body Space or Junction, Body System, Cell Component, Embryonic Structure, Fully Formed Anatomical Structure, Physical Object, Tissue

- **FUNCTION group:** tags related to functions of organisms and substances

  Biologic Function, Cell Function, Chemical Viewed Functionally, Functional Concept, Genetic Function, Organ or Tissue Function, Organism Function, Pathologic Function, Physiologic Function

- **QUALIFIER group:** related to attribute or characteristics of something

  Biomedical or Dental Material, Organism Attribute, Qualitative Concept, Quantitative Concept, Spatial Concept, Temporal Concept

Then, we defined several sequence of the groups, as heuristics. Note that *Temporal Concept* and *Finding* are primitive UMLS tags.

- QUALIFIER + BODYPART
- BODYPART + QUALIFIER
- QUALIFIER + QUALIFIER + BODYPART
- QUALIFIER + FUNCTION + BODYPART
- ACTION + Temporal Concept
- Finding + Temporal Concept

Annotation. For evaluation of our extraction algorithms, we utilized manual annotation of the same texts, by the first author, who is an accredited M.D. The 20 texts included 1368 annotated elements in total. For an annotated element, average number of corresponding MetaMap phrases was 1.46 with standard deviation 1.22.

During the annotation phase, we found that human annotation tends to contain many phrases. For example, "homogeneous eosinophilic masses which form elongated tapered rods up to 30 microns in length, which are scattered throughout the cortex and white matter and are most numerous in the subpial, perivascular and subependymal regions" (OMIM 203450) is annotated as one element. This is the longest of all, which spans 18 MetaMap phrases. This happens because, for annotators with domain knowledge, the set of phrases carries a meaningful information as a symptom, and the phrases are inseparable, although MetaMap segments the phrases in an opposite way.

3   Result

Table 1 shows the performance of the algorithm, in the number of matches against the manual annotation. Baseline indicates the algorithm that uses only *SYMPTOM* tag. Exact (match), Parial (match), and Not Found, is explained

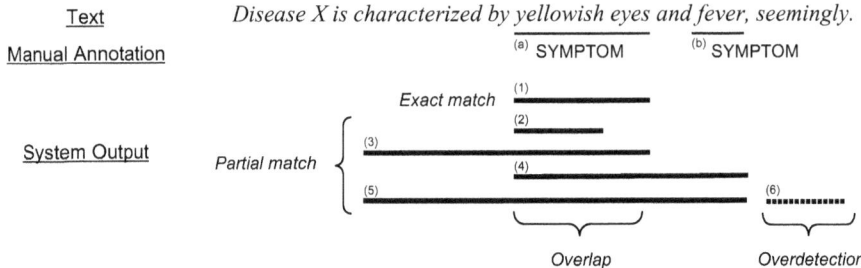

Fig. 2. Definition of Exact, Partial, Overlap, and Overdetection

in Figure 2. For symptom (a), system output (1) is the exact match, which was 13.7% in Table 1. Partial match refers to the cases (2-5), which was 68.4%. Not Found is the number of symptoms in the annotated text that do not have corresponding system output, which was 17.8%. By taking the partial match as success, the algorithm achieved 82.1% Recall (13.7 + 68.4),

The next column applies the heuristics, which works inside the MetaMap phrase boundary (Heuristics 1). The resulting 14.8% exact match and 72.1% partial match sum up to 86.9%, which is a 4.8% increase in the performance. The last column applies the heuristics, beyond the MetaMap phrase boundary (Heuristics 2). This strategy also boosts the performance, which is 89.0%, a 6.9% increase against the baseline.

As Table 1 indicates, the heuristics boost detection performance. However, the heuristics may also increase overdetection (case 6 in Figure 2). To assess the impact, we counted the number of system outputs that have corresponding annotated elements, which is shown in Table 2. In the baseline case, 64.0% of the system output had corresponding annotation, which is *overlap* in Figure 2. On the other hand, 36.1% had no such relationship. And, the heuristics did not affect the ratio of *overdetection*.

Table 1. Performance of detecting symptomatic expressions

Baseline			Baseline + Heuristics 1			Baseline + Heuristics 1 & 2		
Exact	Partial	Not Found	Exact	Partial	Not Found	Exact	Partial	Not Found
188	936	244	202	986	180	226	992	150
(13.7%)	(68.4%)	(17.8%)	(14.8%)	(72.1%)	(13.2%)	(16.5%)	(72.5%)	(11.0%)

Table 2. Amount of Overdetection (OL: Overlap, OD: Overdetection)

Baseline			Baseline + Heuristics 1			Baseline + Heuristics 1 & 2		
# phrases	OL	OD	# phrases	OL	OD	# phrases	OL	OD
1821	1165	657	1945	1244	701	2075	1333	743
	(64.0%)	(36.1%)		(64.0%)	(36.0%)		(64.2%)	(35.8%)

4   Discussion

The result, 89.0% recall, was satisfactory, as a current NLP (Natural Language Processing) tool, although the rate of overdetection reached 36%. Nevertheless, if the system output is later reviewed by domain experts for reliability, the overdetection can be excluded in the post-processing phase. Accordingly, the detection algorithm should be optimized for recall performance. And, to further improve the performance, we analyzed the Not Found cases (150 annotated elements in Table 1) in far more detail.

First of all, there were cases where MetaMap failed to assign UMLS categories that our algorithms depend upon. Unfortunately, MetaMap failed to capture an acronym, *RDS (respiratory distress syndrome)* in OMIM 267450, which happened 17 times. There were 8 other cases where MetaMap failed to interpret simple technical terms, and 3 other cases where MetaMap did not recognize technical adjective of the form *XXX-like* (e.g. *butterfly-like vertebrae* in OMIM 118450), which require morphological analysis. MetaMap also failed to recognize non-technical modifiers, like *few* and *tall*, as Qualitative- or Quantitative-Concept.

Second, there were cases where unexpected UMLS categories were assigned. For example, *axillary sweating*(181450) is expected to be a finding, or a function of the body, but MetaMap assigned a controlled term *Axillary sweat (Sweat of axilla)* in UMLS category *Body Substance*.

Third, MetaMap failed to recognize several abnormal signs, as such. Suppose that substance A is not found in a normal pathological study. Clearly, substance A in a report indicates pathological abnormality of a disease in question. However, UMLS classification does not carry such semantic information, and, categorizes the substance as just another instance in the substance category. Consequently, MetaMap fails to capture the finding. An illustration was *Rosenthal fiber* (Cell Component) in OMIM 203450, which does not exist in a normal cell. Similar problem happens for abnormal findings, if UMLS categorizes them neutrally into, e.g., Functional Concept or Qualifier.

Fourth, combination of *QUALIFIER* and categories like *Body substance*, *Laboratory Procedure* and *Diagnostic Procedure* could have captured descriptions of laboratory test results.

Lastly, there are cases that are beyond the scope of MetaMap tagging. For example, expressions, *The anus was stenotic* (OMIM 248450), and *melanocyte maturation appeared abnormal*(OMIM 211450) clearly indicate symptoms, and can be considered as syntactic variations of *stenotic anus* and *abnormal melanocyte maturation*, respectively. Thus, if *QUALIFIER+BODYPART* pattern is effective, so would be the patten *BODYPART (was|appeared) QUALIFIER*, or more generally *BODYPART VERB QUALIFIER*. Nevertheless, MetaMap does not provide a parser mechanism to interpret the verbal expressions. These cases necessitate other linguistic tools or lexicons, as pursued in [7] and [11]. This applies also to descriptions of test results, e.g. *hCG stimulation tests showed normal testosterone responses* (OMIM 181450).

5   Related Works

Extraction of symptom expression in a text was first investigated as a method for automated analysis of medical literature [18]. They used Xerox tagger to extract noun phrases, and use heuristic rules on UMLS semantic categories assigned to the words in the phrases and existence of adjectives or numerals. For example, the sentence *Eight demented cases had absent neocortical neurofibrillary tangles* is extracted as describing findings because of *neurofibrillary tangles* which has Cell Component type and an adjective *absent*. Their result is comparable to ours (precision 65 % and recall 82 %). This work lead to research for mapping of expressions in a text and their associated concept [2,15,1], which furnished the basis for our study. Our approach is similar to this work [18], in grouping UMLS semantic categories into broader concepts and in applying heuristics to the concept groups to gain recall. We differ in that the proposed scheme uses only MetaMap and utilizes group sequences as heuristics. Equivalent effect of using adjectives is achieved by using QUALIFIER group of UMLS concepts in our heuristics, though some adjectives which were not assigned UMLS categories (e.g., *few*, *tall*) are ignored.

MetaMap has been used for many medical NLP projects, and its output has been evaluated extensively [6,8,16]. There are also a series of researches that exploited MetaMap for improved accuracy through extension [3,13] and through modification of the system [9,17].

There are systems for extracting phenotype information from OMIM Clinical Synopsis section, where the typical symptoms and signs for the disease is structured in a table [7,5]. We use the free-text description, not the Clinical Synopsis, in OMIM, simply because our target is description of disease in general. We used OMIM as a text database, and structured description of a disease is less likely to be available in a medical literature.

Cohen et al. [7] describes a system for extracting phenotype from the OMIM Clinical Synopsis. They combine MetaMap and a CFG parser to cluster the expressions for similar phenotype, and negation extraction to decrease the false positive results. Cantor and Lussier [5] also extracts phenotype from Clinical Synopsis, and performs text processing to normalize the variants of names, but the detail of their text analysis is not described in the paper.

In reference [11], disease named entities are extracted from OMIM free text by dictionary lookup, statistical learning, and MetaMap, but direct comparison is difficult because our purpose is also to extract symptoms and findings, which have often more complex structure (i.e. verb phrases, sentences) than named entities.

6   Conclusion

In this paper, we presented a lightweight approach to build a disease knowledge base for diagnostic decision support systems, utilizing MetaMap. The UMLS semantic tags in MetaMap output achieved 82% recall and 64% precision, and simple heuristics for interpretation contributed additional 7%, in the extraction of symptomatic expressions in descriptions of diseases.

Because the resulting data might include failures and might have excluded important relationship, manual verification is preferable. Nevertheless, the automated generation of the relation data would reduce the total cost for building a disease knowledge base, by providing a foundation for the human intervention.

Our future work has four possible directions. First, we may investigate on the further performance boost of the extraction algorithm, as suggested by the failure analysis. Second, coding of symptomatic expressions, against the symptom master, or representation of the clinical knowledge with a standardized terminology, is needed. Third, it would be beneficial to expand the inputs, onto various sources, not limited to OMIM. Lastly, efficient tools for manual verification must be provided.

Acknowledgment. We are grateful to Mr. Kazuaki Tanida at University of Tokyo for preprocessing of OMIM data, Mr. Maiki Nonaka who performed preliminary study of the heuristics at Kogakuin University, and Dr. Junichi Tsujii gave us useful suggestions for the work, including the MetaMap utilization. Dr. Takatoshi Ishikawa helped us in the early phase of the study, for OMIM annotation.

References

1. Aronson, A.R.: Effective mapping of biomedical text to the UMLS Metathesaurus: the MetaMap program. In: AMIA Annual Symposium, pp. 17–21 (2001)
2. Aronson, A.R., Lang, F.M.: An overview of MetaMap: historical perspective and recent advances. Journal of the American Medical Informatics Association 17(3), 229–236 (2010)
3. Bashyam, V., Divita, G., Bennett, D.B., Browne, A.C., Taira, R.K.: A normalized lexical lookup approach to identifying UMLS concepts in free text. Studies in Health Technology and Informatics 129(Pt 1), 545–549 (2007)
4. Bodenreider, O.: The unified medical language system (UMLS): integrating biomedical terminology. Nucleic Acids Research 32(Database issue), D267–D270 (2004)
5. Cantor, M.N., Lussier, Y.A.: Mining OMIM for insight into complex diseases. Studies in Health Technology and Informatics 107(Pt 2), 753–757 (2004)
6. Chapman, W.W., Fiszman, M., Dowling, J.N., Chapman, B.E., Rindflesch, T.C.: Identifying respiratory findings in emergency department reports for biosurveillance using MetaMap. Studies in Health Technology and Informatics 107(Pt 1), 487–491 (2004)
7. Cohen, R., Gefen, A., Elhadad, M., Birk, O.S.: CSI-OMIM–Clinical Synopsis Search in OMIM. BMC Bioinformatics 12, 65 (2011)
8. Divita, G., Tse, T., Roth, L.: Failure analysis of MetaMap Transfer (MMTx). Studies in Health Technology and Informatics 107(Pt 2), 763–767 (2004)
9. Gschwandtner, T., Kaiser, K., Martini, P., Miksch, S.: Easing semantically enriched information retrieval-an interactive semi-automatic annotation system for medical documents. International Journal of Human-Computer Studies 68(6), 370–385 (2010)

10. INSERM SC11: Orphanet, `http://www.orpha.net/`
11. Jimeno, A., Jimenez-Ruiz, E., Lee, V., Gaudan, S., Berlanga, R., Rebholz-Schuhmann, D.: Assessment of disease named entity recognition on a corpus of annotated sentences. BMC Bioinformatics 9(suppl. 3), S3 (2008)
12. John Hopkins University: OMIM: Online Mendelian Inheritance in Man, `http://www.ncbi.nlm.nih.gov/omim`
13. Meystre, S., Haug, P.J.: Evaluation of medical problem extraction from electronic clinical documents using MetaMap Transfer (MMTx). Studies in Health Technology and Informatics 116, 823–828 (2005)
14. Miller, R.A.: Computer-assisted diagnostic decision support: history, challenges, and possible paths forward. Adv. in Health Sci. Educ. 14, 89–106 (2009)
15. Osborne, J.D., Lin, S., Zhu, L., Kibbe, W.A.: Mining biomedical data using MetaMap Transfer (MMTx) and the Unified Medical Language System (UMLS). Methods in Molecular Biology 408, 153–169 (2007)
16. Pratt, W., Yetisgen-Yildiz, M.: A study of biomedical concept identification: MetaMap vs. people. In: AMIA Annual Symposium, pp. 529–533 (2003)
17. Segura-Bedmar, I., Martinez, P., Segura-Bedmar, M.: Drug name recognition and classification in biomedical texts. a case study outlining approaches underpinning automated systems. Drug Discovery Today 13(17-18), 816–823 (2008)
18. Sneiderman, C.A., Rindflesch, T.C., Aronson, A.R.: Finding the findings: identification of findings in medical literature using restricted natural language processing. In: AMIA Annual Fall Symposium, pp. 239–243 (1996)

Novel Hybrid Feature Selection Algorithms for Diagnosing Erythemato-Squamous Diseases

Juanying Xie[1,2], Jinhu Lei[1], Weixin Xie[2,3], Xinbo Gao[2],
Yong Shi[4], and Xiaohui Liu[5]

[1] School of computer science, Shaanxi Normal University, Xi'an 710062, China
[2] School of Electronic Engineering, Xidian University, Xi'an 710071, China
[3] School of Information Engineering, Shenzhen University, Shenzhen 518060, China
[4] CAS Research Centre of Fictitious Economy and Data Science,
Chinese Academy of Sciences, Beijing 100080, China
[5] School of Information systems, Computing and Mathematics, Brunel University,
London UB8 3PH, UK

Abstract. This paper proposes hybrid feature selection algorithms to build the efficient diagnostic models based on a new accuracy criterion, generalized F-score (GF) and SVM. The hybrid algorithms adopt Sequential Forward Search (SFS), and Sequential Forward Floating Search (SFFS), and Sequential Backward Floating Search (SBFS), respectively, with SVM to accomplish hybrid feature selection with the new accuracy criterion to guide the procedure. We call them as modified GFSFS, GFSFFS and GFSBFS, respectively. These hybrid methods combine the advantages of filters and wrappers to select the optimal feature subset from the original feature set to build the efficient classifiers. To get the best and statistically meaningful classifiers, we not only conduct 10-fold cross validation experiments on training subset, but also on the whole erythemato-squamous diseases datasets. Experimental results show that our proposed hybrid methods construct efficient diagnosis classifiers with high average accuracy when compared with traditional algorithms.

Keywords: generalized F-score, Support Vector Machines, Feature Selection, Sequential Forward Search, Sequential Forward Floating Search, Sequential Backward Floating Search, Erythemato-squamous Diseases.

1 Introduction

Erythemato-squamous diseases are frequently seen in outpatient dermatology departments [1, 2]. There are six groups of the diseases. They are psoriasis, seboreic dermatitis, lichen planus, pityriasis rosea, chronic dermatitis and pityriasis rubra pilaris. All of them share the clinical features of erythema with very few differences. This makes it very challenging to perform a differential diagnosis for erythemato-squamous diseases in dermatology.

A biopsy is necessary for diagnosing these diseases, while unfortunately they share many histopathological features. Another difficulty for the differential diagnosis is that one disease may show features of another at the initial stage and

J. He et al. (Eds.): HIS 2012, LNCS 7231, pp. 173–185, 2012.
© Springer-Verlag Berlin Heidelberg 2012

display its own characteristic features at the following stages. Patients were first evaluated clinically with 12 features. Afterwards, skin samples were taken for evaluation with 22 histopathological features. The values of these features are determined by an analysis of the samples under a microscope [1].

Many experts devote themselves to studying the diagnoses of erythemato-squamous diseases, and there has been much work in the area. These works mainly involve studying the efficiency of different machine learning methods to diagnose erythemato-squamous diseases and aim to uncover an optimal way to determine the type of erythemato-squamous disease according to its features [3–10]. Recently, there are clustering based methods to diagnose erythemato-squamous diseases [11].

The common character of above works is that they apply different approaches directly to the problem without feature selection. Feature selections for classification will preserve the important features for building an efficient classifier and remove the noisy and redundant ones, so that the classification rules will become concise and the classification accuracy will be improved. In diagnostic area some features are necessary to make a correct decision, while others may be redundant and affect the doctor to make a right diagnostic decision. So it is necessary to study and discover an efficient feature selection method to delete the noisy or redundant features and preserve the necessary ones, so that to help doctors to make a sound diagnostic decision.

In this connection, Liu *et al* [12] proposed a feature selection algorithm with dynamic mutual information, and adopted four typical classifiers to study the diagnoses of erythemato-squamous diseases. In addition, Karabatak and Ince [13] proposed another feature selection method based on association rules and neural network. Xie *et al* [14, 15] suggested efficient feature selection methods to diagnose the diseases.

While our previous work has the disadvantage that the accuracy criterion we used to evaluate the performance of temporary SVM classifier to guide feature selection procedure may lead the classifier to lean to one group of erythemato-squamous diseases. For example, if we face to classify a binary classification problem, and there are 90 samples in the first group, and 10 in the second group. Under this condition, if all samples are classified to the first class and none to the second class, then the accuracy is 90%. This is the situation we should avoid because the whole samples in the second class are misclassified. To overcome this kind of potential disadvantage we modified the definition of accuracy and propose several new hybrid feature selection algorithms in this paper. Experiments are conducted to demonstrate that our new hybrid feature selection algorithms are valid in building efficient classifiers for diagnosing erythemato-squamous diseases.

This paper is organized as follows. Section 2 describes the principal feature selection method and our hybrid feature selection algorithms. Section 3 demonstrates our experimental results and analyzes them in detail. Finally, section 4 draws conclusions and describes the future work.

2   Hybrid Feature Selection Algorithms

Feature selection plays an important role in building a classification system [16–18]. It not only reduces the dimensionality of data, but also reduces the computational cost and gains a good classification performance.

The general feature selection algorithms comprise two categories: the filter and wrapper methods [19, 20]. The filter methods identify a feature subset from original ones with a given evaluation criterion which is independent of learning algorithms. While the wrappers choose those features with high prediction performance estimated by a specified learning algorithm. The filters are efficient because of its independence to learning algorithms, while wrappers can obtain higher classification accuracy with the deficiency in generalization and computational cost. So many experts focus on study the hybrid feature selection methods recently. Hybrid feature selection methods combine the advantages of filters and wrappers to uncover high quality classifiers.

In this paper, we present several hybrid feature selection algorithms that adopt the generalized F-score to rank features. We extend SFS and SFFS and SBFS to select the necessary features while SVM with our modified accuracy as the criterion to evaluate the performance of the corresponding SVM to guide the feature selection procedure.

2.1   Generalized F-Score

The original F-score is used to measure the discrimination of two sets of real numbers [18]. We generalized it in [14] to measure the discrimination between more than two sets of real numbers. Here are the definitions of the generalized F-score. Given training vectors x_k, $k = 1, 2, \cdots, m$, and the number of subsets $l(l \geq 2)$, if the size of the jth subset is n_j, $j = 1, 2, \cdots, l$, then the F-score of the ith feature is F_i.

$$
F_i = \frac{\sum\limits_{j=1}^{l} (\bar{x}_i^{(j)} - \bar{x}_i)^2}{\sum\limits_{j=1}^{l} \frac{1}{n_j-1} \sum\limits_{k=1}^{n_j} (x_{k,i}^{(j)} - \bar{x}_i^{(j)})^2}
\tag{1}
$$

where $\bar{x}_i$ and $\bar{x}_i^{(j)}$ are the average of the ith feature of the whole dataset and the jth subset respectively, and $x_{k,i}^{(j)}$ is the ith feature of the kth instance in the jth subset. The numerator of (1) indicates the discrimination between each subset, and denominator the one within each subset. The larger the F-score is, the more likely this feature is discriminative.

2.2   The Modified Classification Accuracy

The accuracy of a classifier is often used to evaluate the performance of it. The accuracy is often defined as that in the equation (2).

$$
accuracy = \frac{N_r}{N}
\tag{2}
$$

where N_r is the number of samples which are classified correctly, and N the total number of samples which are to be classified. This accuracy does not consider the performance of a classifier on each class, which sometimes will lead the skew on some classes. For example, there is a cancer diagnostic problem with 90 no cancer patient and 10 cancer patient. Now we have got a classifier that can recognize all no cancer patient and zero cancer patients. Although the accuracy of the classifier is 90%, it is not a good classifier. So we define a new accuracy in the equation (3).

$$new\_accuracy = \frac{1}{l} \sum_{c=1}^{l} \frac{N_r^c}{N^c} \tag{3}$$

where l is the number of classes which are classified in a problem, the N_r^c is the number of samples which are correctly classified in the cth class, and N^c is the total number of samples which are to be classified in the cth class. This new accuracy does consider the performance of a classifier on each class that is considering in the classification problem to overcome the skew of the old one's.

2.3 Several Hybrid Feature Selection Algorithms

The popular feature selection strategies include sequential forward search (SFS) [21] and sequential backward search (SBS) [22] and sequential forward floating search (SFFS) and sequential backward floating search (SBFS) [23].

Here we extend the traditional SFS, SFFS, and SBFS strategies. We first rank features according their F-score, then deal with them one by one. In SFS, we add features according to their rank order, not as the traditional SFS which considers that the added feature must be the best one when combined with the selected ones. In SFFS, we test the feature to be added, if the new accuracy of the temporary classifier goes up then add it, otherwise do not add it. In SBFS, the procedure starts with all feature are included, each iteration we test deleting the current lowest rank feature, if the accuracy of the temporary classifier becomes worse, then do not delete the feature, otherwise delete it. These procedures continue until all features are tested.

In order to get the optimal model, we adopt grid search technique and 10-fold cross validation experiments on training subsets to discover the best parameter pairs (C, γ) for RBF, so that we can get the separating hyperplane with the largest margin. The range of C and γ we considering are $log_2 C = \{-5, -4, -3, \cdots, 13, 14, 15\}$ and $log_2 \gamma = \{-15, -13, -11, \cdots, 3, 1, 3\}$, respectively.

Here we present three hybrid feature selection algorithms, named modified GFSFS, GFSFFS and GFSBFS, respectively. The generalized F-score plays the role of filters, and our extend SFS and SFFS and SBFS, respectively, with SVM and our modified accuracy act as wrappers. Via modified GFSFS and GFSFFS and GFSBFS we select necessary features and eliminated redundant ones, so that we construct a sound predictor in diagnosing erythemato-squamous diseases.

The pseudo code of our modified GFSFS is here.

step 1: Determine the training and testing subsets of exemplars; Initialize the selected-feature-subset empty, and selecting-feature-subset with all features;

step 2: Computing the F-score value for each feature according to the training subset, and sort features in descending order according to their F-score;

step 3: Add the top one feature of the selecting-feature-subset to selected-feature-subset, and deleted the selected feature from selecting-feature-subset as well;

step 4: Train the training subset with feature in selected-feature-subset to construct the temporary optimal SVM classifier, the optimal parameters of the SVM are determined via grid search technique with 10-fold cross validation described above;

step 5: Classify exemplars in testing subsets with feature in selected-feature-subset and record the testing accuracy;

step 6: go to step 3, until the selecting-feature-subset becomes empty;

Although our modified GFSFS can get a comparable high performance in diagnosing erythemato-squamous diseases, it may suffer the possible feature subset "nesting" weakness that is the nature of SFS. The coming hybrid feature selection algorithm, modified GFSFFS, will overcome this disadvantage of our modified GFSFS by considering the correlation between features, so once the modified accuracy of the temporary classifier on training subset cannot go up, then the added feature will be deleted from selected-feature-subset. The details of our modified GFSFFS are as followings.

Step 1: Compute the F-score for each feature via generalized F-score on this fold training subset, and sort features in descending order according to their F-score; Initialize the selected-feature-subset empty and the selecting-feature-subset all features;

Step 2: Delete the top feature in selecting-feature-subset and add it to selected-feature-subset;

Step 3: Train the training subset to build the optimal predictor model where the optimal parameter for the kernel function of SVM is determined by the grid search technique and 10-fold cross-validation described above;

Step 4: If the modified accuracy of training subset is not improved, then the feature that has just been added will be eliminated from the selected-feature-subset;

Step 5: Go to Step 2 till all features in selecting-feature-subset have been processed.

The features in the selected-feature-subset comprise the best feature subset of this fold, and the last SVM classifier is the optimal diagnostic model we are looking for.

To further prove the efficiency of our modified accuracy, we propose modified GFSBFS hybrid feature selection algorithm and describe its procedure here.

Step 1: Compute the F-score for each feature via generalized F-score on this fold training subset, and sort features in descending order according to their F-score; Initialize the selected-feature-subset with all features, and the visited tag for each feature unvisited;

Step 2: Train the training subset to build the optimal predictor model where the optimal parameter for the kernel function of SVM is determined by the grid search technique and 10-fold cross validation described above; Record the accuracy of the model on training subset in our modified accuracy;

Step 3: Delete the last unvisited feature in selected-feature-subset, and let the visited tag of this feature be visited;

Step 4: Train the training subset to build the optimal predictor model where the optimal parameter for the kernel function of SVM is determined in the approach described above; Record the accuracy of the model on training subset in the modified accuracy;

Step 5: If the accuracy of training subset does not go up, keep the feature that it has just been deleted back to selected-feature-subset;

Step 6: Go to Step 3, until all features in selected-feature-subset have been visited.

At last those features left in selected-feature-subset are the necessary ones to build the best diagnostic model for this fold.

3 Experiments and Analysis

In this section, we demonstrate the experimental results we obtained on the erythemato-squamous diseases dataset from UCI machine learning repository in detail, and analyze the results in depth.

Our aim is to construct an optimal diagnostic model to determine the type of erythemato-squamous disease according to its features. In order to get the sound and statistically classifier we did 10-fold cross validation experiments on the datasets. We repeated choosing the ith sample from each class to construct the ith fold, until each sample is chosen. We chose one fold as testing subset, and the other nine folds as training subset, then calculated the F-score of each feature on training subset. After that we use our modified GFSFS, GFSFFS and GFSBFS, respectively, and SVM with our modified accuracy criterion to construct the optimal diagnostic models. This procedure is iterated until each fold being chosen as testing subset.

We did our experiment using the library of SVM provided by Chang & Lin. As a comparison we demonstrate the experimental results of the corresponding algorithms that use the unmodified accuracy as the criterion to evaluate the SVM classifiers to guild feature selection procedures. Table 1 and 2 demonstrate the

Table 1. Experimental results of GFSFS on eryrhenato-squamous diseases dataset with unmodified accuracy

fold	selected feature subset	number of selected features	classification accuracy(%)
1	33, 27,29, 31, 6, 12, 20, 15, 25, 22, 8, 7, 21, 30, 9, 10, 16, 24, 28, 14, 5, 26	22	100.0000
2	33, 29, 27, 31, 6, 12, 15, 20, 25, 22, 7, 8, 21, 30, 9, 24, 10, 28, 16, 14, 5, 26	22	97.2222
3	33, 27, 31, 29, 6, 12, 22, 25, 15, 20, 8, 7, 30, 21, 9, 28, 10, 16, 24, 14, 5, 34, 26	23	100.0000
4	33, 27, 31, 29, 6, 12, 20, 15, 22, 7, 25, 8, 21, 30, 9, 28, 16, 24, 10, 14, 5, 34, 26	23	94.4444
5	33, 27, 6, 31, 29, 12, 15, 22, 20, 25, 7, 8, 21, 30, 9, 28, 24, 16, 10, 14, 5	21	100.0000
6	27, 33, 31, 6, 29, 12, 25?22, 15, 20, 7, 8, 21, 30, 9, 24, 16, 28, 10, 14, 5, 34, 26	23	100.0000
7	33, 27, 31, 29, 6, 12, 20, 15, 22, 7, 25, 8, 21, 30, 9, 24, 28, 16, 10, 14, 5	21	100.0000
8	33, 27, 29, 12, 31, 6, 15, 22, 20, 7, 25, 8, 21, 30, 9, 28, 16, 24, 10, 14, 5, 34,26	23	97.2222
9	33, 27, 29, 31, 6, 12, 22, 20, 25, 15, 7, 8, 21, 30, 9, 28, 16, 24, 10, 14, 5, 34, 26	23	100.0000
10	33, 27, 31, 29, 6, 12, 20, 22, 15, 25, 8, 7, 21, 30, 9, 28, 10, 24, 16, 14, 5	21	100.0000
average & common	33, 27, 29, 31, 6, 12, 20, 15, 25, 22, 8, 7, 21, 30, 9, 10, 16, 24, 28, 14, 5	22.20	98.89

results of 10-fold cross validation experiment of GFSFS and modified GFSFS, respectively. Table 3 and 4 show the results of 10-fold cross validation experiment of GFSFFS and modified GFSFFS, respectively. The 10-fold cross validation experimental results of GFSBFS and modified GFSBFS are listed in Table 5 and 6. Table 7 summarizes the classification accuracies of all available methods.

From the figures in Table 1 and 2 we can see that our new hybrid feature selection algorithm, modified GFSFS has got better classification accuracy of 99.17% than the corresponding GFSFS with traditional accuracy criterion. The accuracy of later is 98.89%. The selected features and test accuracy in each fold are nearly same except that in the fold eight. In this fold, our new GFSFS has got the 100% classification accuracy with 21 features, while the other GFSFS only gets 97.22% accuracy, and the selected feature subset is bigger than that of our modified GFSFS with two more features. The average size of selected feature subset of our new GFSFS is smaller than that of the corresponding GFSFS. The common selected features of these two algorithms are similar.

Table 3 and 4 tell us that our modified GFSFFS not only improves the classification accuracy from 96.08% to 98.33% compared to the GFSFFS with traditional accuracy, but also reduces the dimension of dataset greatly. The size

Table 2. Experimental results of GFSFS on eryrhenato-squamous diseases dataset with modified accuracy

fold	selected feature subset	number of selected features	classification accuracy(%)
1	33, 27, 29, 31, 6, 12, 20, 15, 25, 22, 8, 7, 21, 30, 9, 10, 16, 24, 28, 14, 5, 26	22	100.0000
2	33, 29, 27, 31, 6, 12, 15, 20, 25, 22, 7, 8, 21, 30, 9, 24, 10, 28, 16, 14, 5, 26	22	97.2222
3	33, 27, 31, 29, 6, 12, 22, 25, 15, 20, 8, 7, 30, 21, 9, 28, 10, 16, 24, 14, 5, 34, 26	23	100.0000
4	33, 27, 31, 29, 6, 12, 20, 15, 22, 7, 25, 8, 21, 30, 9, 28, 16, 24, 10, 14, 5, 34, 26	23	94.4444
5	33, 27, 6, 31, 29, 12, 15, 22, 20, 25, 7, 8, 21, 30, 9, 28, 24, 16, 10, 14, 5	21	100.0000
6	27, 33, 31, 6, 29, 12, 25?22, 15, 20, 7, 8, 21, 30, 9, 24, 16, 28, 10, 14, 5, 34, 26	23	100.0000
7	33, 27, 31, 29, 6, 12, 20, 15, 22, 7, 25, 8, 21, 30, 9, 24, 28, 16, 10, 14, 5	21	100.0000
8	33, 27, 29, 12, 31, 6, 15, 22, 20, 7, 25, 8, 21, 30, 9, 28, 16, 24, 10, 14, 5	21	100.0000
9	33, 27, 29, 31, 6, 12, 22, 20, 25, 15, 7, 8, 21, 30, 9, 28, 16, 24, 10, 14, 5, 34, 26	23	100.0000
10	33, 27, 31, 29, 6, 12, 20, 22, 15, 25, 8, 7, 21, 30, 9, 28, 10, 24, 16, 14, 5	21	100.0000
average & common	33, 27, 29, 31, 6, 12, 20, 15, 25, 22, 8, 7, 21, 30, 9, 10, 16, 24, 28, 14, 5	22	99.17

Table 3. Experimental results of GFSFFS on eryrhenato-squamous diseases dataset with unmodified accuracy

fold	selected feature subset	number of selected features	classification accuracy(%)
1	7, 31, 9, 5, 34, 4, 14, 28, 15, 17, 26, 25	12	100
2	5, 7, 14, 9, 31, 28, 15, 21, 16, 1, 17, 33, 18, 13	14	91.6667
3	26, 7, 31, 28, 9, 34, 15, 21, 14, 5, 2, 4, 17	13	100
4	7, 31, 30, 9, 5, 34, 28, 15, 21, 16, 4, 14, 1, 25, 33	15	88.8889
5	7, 31, 28, 15, 21, 5, 4, 14, 9, 34, 33, 29, 26, 18, 17	15	97.2222
6	7, 31, 9, 34, 28, 15, 21, 14, 16, 5, 33, 27, 26	13	97.2222
7	7, 31, 28, 9, 15, 21, 16, 14, 5, 4, 2, 33, 25	13	94.4444
8	7, 31, 33, 5, 28, 21, 15, 26, 29	9	97.2222
9	7, 31, 9, 34, 28, 21, 15, 5, 16, 14, 4, 2, 26, 17	14	94.1176
10	7, 31, 9, 28, 34, 15, 21, 5, 16, 4, 1, 18, 33, 32, 13	15	100
average & common	7, 31, 5, 28, 15	13.3	96.08

Table 4. Experimental results of GFSFFS on eryrhenato-squamous diseases dataset with modified accuracy

fold	selected feature subset	number of selected features	classification accuracy(%)
1	33, 29, 31, 6, 20, 15, 7, 21, 10, 16, 28, 14, 5, 26, 18	15	100.0000
2	33, 29, 31, 15, 20, 22, 7, 28, 16, 14, 5, 26, 18	13	94.4444
3	33, 31, 6, 22, 25, 15, 20, 7, 28, 10, 16, 14, 5, 26	14	100.0000
4	33, 31, 6, 20, 15, 7, 25, 21, 9, 28, 24, 14, 5, 26, 19	15	94.4444
5	33, 6, 31, 15, 22, 20, 25, 28, 16, 10, 14, 5, 4, 26	14	100.0000
6	27, 31, 22, 15, 20, 7, 16, 10, 14, 5, 26	11	97.2222
7	33, 31, 6, 20, 15, 22, 25, 28, 16, 10, 14, 5, 26, 18	14	100.0000
8	33, 29, 31, 6, 15, 22, 20, 16, 14, 5, 26	11	97.2222
9	33, 29, 31, 6, 22, 15, 9, 28, 16, 10, 14, 5, 26	13	100.0000
10	33, 31, 20, 15, 7, 21, 9, 28, 10, 14, 5, 26	12	100.0000
average & common	31, 15, 14, 5, 26	13.2	98.33

Table 5. Experimental results of GFSBFS on eryrhenato-squamous diseases dataset with unmodified accuracy

fold	selected feature subset	number of selected features	classification accuracy(%)
1	17, 13, 19, 2, 3, 4, 34, 26, 5, 14, 28, 16, 15, 33	14	94.7368
2	32, 18, 13, 17, 1, 26, 5, 14, 28, 15, 31, 29	12	94.4444
3	32, 18, 17, 13, 1, 19, 3, 23, 4, 26, 34, 5, 14, 16, 28, 9, 15, 33	18	100
4	32, 13, 17, 1, 19, 2, 3, 23, 4, 26, 34, 5,14, 9, 7, 22, 15, 31, 33	19	97.2222
5	1, 13, 17, 19, 2, 23, 26, 14, 24, 28, 9, 7, 25, 22, 15, 33	16	94.4444
6	32, 18, 1, 13, 17, 19, 2, 3, 4, 26, 5, 28, 9, 15, 31, 27	16	91.6667
7	32, 13, 18, 1, 17, 19, 2, 11, 4, 23, 3, 26, 34, 5, 14, 10, 16, 28, 24, 9, 30, 21, 8, 25, 7, 22, 15, 20, 12, 6, 29, 31, 27, 33	34	97.2222
8	32, 17, 13, 1, 3, 26, 5, 9, 30, 20, 22, 15, 31, 33	14	97.2222
9	18, 13, 17, 1, 19, 2, 23, 3, 4, 26, 5, 14, 28, 15, 31, 33	16	97.0588
10	32, 18, 13, 17, 1, 19, 11, 2, 3, 4, 23, 26, 34, 5, 14, 16, 24, 10, 28, 9, 30, 21, 7, 8, 25, 15,22, 20, 12, 6, 29, 31, 27, 33	34	94.1176
average & common	17,13, 26, 15	19.3	95.81

Table 6. Experimental results of GFSBFS on eryrhenato-squamous diseases dataset with modified accuracy

fold	selected feature subset	number of selected features	classification accuracy(%)
1	13, 1, 19, 2, 4, 23, 34, 26, 5, 14, 28, 16, 7, 15, 33	15	97.36842105
2	18, 13, 17, 19, 2, 3, 4, 23, 26, 5, 16, 28, 9, 22, 31, 33	16	94.44444444
3	32, 18, 17, 13, 1, 19, 23, 4, 26, 34, 5, 14, 28, 9, 3 7, 15, 33	18	94.44444444
4	32, 18, 13, 17, 19, 2, 3, 4, 26, 34, 5, 14, 16, 28, 7, 15, 20, 33	18	97.22222222
5	1, 13, 17, 2, 3, 26, 4, 5, 28, 9, 7, 15, 33	13	94.44444444
6	18, 1, 13, 17, 2, 3, 4, 23, 26, 34, 5, 14, 28, 16, 15, 22, 31, 27	18	91.66666667
7	13, 18, 1, 17, 23, 26, 34, 5, 14, 16, 7, 22, 15, 20, 27, 33	16	97.22222222
8	32, 18, 17, 13, 1, 19, 2, 3, 4, 26, 34, 5, 10, 28, 9, 21, 25, 7, 22, 15, 27	21	88.88888889
9	32, 13, 1, 11, 19, 2, 23, 3, 26, 34, 5, 14, 10, 24, 16, 28, 9, 21, 7, 15, 33	21	97.05882353
10	13, 1, 19, 3, 4, 26, 5, 14, 28, 9, 15, 22, 29, 31, 33	15	100
average & common	13, 26, 5	17.1	95.28

of selected feature subset is about the half of the corresponding GFSFS. The common selected features in modified GFSFFS and corresponding GFSFFS are 5, 15, and 31, which is the subset of the common features of the two GFSFS hybrid feature selection algorithms.

Table 5 and 6 show that the modified GFSBFS algorithm cannot advance the accuracy of the diagnostic model of GFSBFS except causes some extent reduction in dimension. The common features of these two GFSBFS are 13 and 26. Compared to the results of our other hybrid feature algorithms based on the two different forward search strategies, we can say that the backward search strategy is not good.

The feature 5 is the only one common feature in our modified GFSFS and GFSFFS and GFSBFS algorithms. It can be seen that feature 5: Koebner phenomenon is the most important feature to be considered when establishes an efficient diagnostic model.

The summary in Table 7 demonstrates that our hybrid feature selection algorithm, modified GFSFS, combining the modified accuracy and generalized F-score and SVM for diagnosising erythemato-squamous diseases obtains the best result with 99.17% classification accuracy among all studies. The GFSFS follows. Then is the modified GFSFFS, GFSFFS, GFSBFS, and modified GFS-BFS. While considering the size of the selected feature subset, the modified GFSFFS is a comparable one when construct an efficient diagnosing model for erythemato-squamous diseases.

From the above analysis it is clear that we have got the best diagnostic model for diagnosing erythemato-squamous diseases.

Table 7. Classification accuracies of our method and other classifiers from literature

Author	Method	Classification accuracy(%)
Übeyli and Güler (2005)	ANFIS	95.50
Luukka and Leppälampi (2006)	Fuzzy similarity-based classification	97.02
Polat and Günes (2006)	Fuzzy weighted pre-processing	88.18
	K-NN based weighted pre-processing	97.57
	Decision tree	99.00
Nanni (2006)	LSVM	97.22
	RS	97.22
	B1_5	97.50
	B1_10	98.10
	B1_15	97.22
	B2_5	97.50
	B2_10	97.80
	B2_15	98.30
Luukka (2007)	Similarity measure	97.80
Übeyli (2008)	Multiclass SVM with the ECOC	98.32
Polat and Günes (2009)	C4.5 and one-against-all	96.71
Übeylii (2009)	CNN	97.77
Liu et al. (2009)	Naïve Bayes	96.72
	1-NN	92.18
	C4.5	95.08
	PIPPER	92.20
Karabatak and Ince (2009)	AR and NN	98.61
Übeyli and Doğdu (2010)	K-means clustering	94.22
Xie *et al* (2010)	IFSFFS	97.58
Xie *et al* (2011)	IFSFS	98.61
This study	GFSFS	98.89
	modified GFSFS	99.17
	GFSFFS	96.08
	modified GFSFFS	98.33
	GFSBFS	95.81
	modified GFSBFS	95.28

4 Conclusion

This paper proposes a new accuracy definition, and uses it to evaluate the performance of a temporary classifier in several hybrid feature selection algorithms to establish the diagnostic models for diagnosing erythemato-squamous diseases.

The new hybrid feature selection algorithms are based on the generalized F-score and SVM with the new classification accuracy to evaluate the performance of a temporary classifier to guide the feature selection procedure. The new hybrid feature selection algorithms combine the strengths of filters and wrappers to uncover the optimal feature subset with the best diagnostic efficiency.

The results of 10-fold cross validation experiments on erythemato-squamous diseases dataset show that our proposed hybrid feature selection algorithms, modified GFSFS, GFSFFS, and GFSBFS, have obtained the average classification accuracies of 99.17%, 98.33%, and 95.28% with the average size of selected feature subsets of 22, 13.2, and 17.1 respectively. While the classification accuracy of GFSFS, GFSFFS, and GFSBFS are 98.89%, 98.06%, and 95.81%, and the size of selected feature subset of them are 22.2, 13.3, and 19.3 respectively. Considering the results, our hybrid feature selection algorithms are promising ones that can construct the effective diagnostic models for diagnosing erythemato-squamous diseases.

However, in order to get the best model, we performed 10-fold cross validation experiments and grid search technique for the optimal parameters of SVM on training subset, which incurred extra computation costs. Minimizing this cost is one of the directions for our future work.

Acknowledgments. We are most grateful to Dr H. Altay Guvenir who donated the erythemato-squamous dataset as well as to C. C. Chang and C. J. Lin who provide the helpful SVM toolbox. This work is supported in part by the grant of the Fundamental Research Funds for the Central Universities of GK200901006 and GK201001003 in PR China, and is also supported by the Natural Science Basic Research Plan in Shaanxi Province of PR China (Program No. 2010JM3004), and by the Chinese Academy of Sciences under Innovative Group Overseas Partnership Grant and National Natural Science Foundation of China Major International Joint Research Project (NO.71110107026).

References

1. Güvenir, H.A., Demiröz, G., İlter, N.: Learning differential diagnosis of erythemato-squamous diseases using voting feature intervals. Artificial Intelligence in Medicine 13, 147–165 (1998)
2. Güvenir, H.A., Emeksiz, N.: An expert system for the differential diagnosis of erythemato-squamous diseases. Expert Systems with Applications 18, 43–49 (2000)
3. Übeyli, E.D., Güler, İ.: Automatic detection of erythemato-squamous diseases using adaptive neuro-fuzzy inference systems. Computers in Biology and Medicine 35, 421–433 (2005)
4. Luukka, P., Leppälampi, T.: Similarity classifier with generalized mean applied to medical data. Computers in Biology and Medicine 36, 1026–1040 (2006)
5. Polat, K., Güneş, S.: The effect to diagnostic accuracy of decision tree classifier of fuzzy and k-NN based weighted pre-processing methods to diagnosis of erythemato-squamous diseases. Digital Signal Processing 16, 922–930 (2006)
6. Nanni, L.: An ensemble of classifiers for the diagnosis of erythemato-squamous diseases. Neurocomputing 69, 842–845 (2006)
7. Luukka, P.: Similarity classifier using similarity measure derived from Yu's norms in classification of medical data sets. Computers in Biology and Medicine 37, 1133–1140 (2007)
8. Übeyli, E.D.: Multiclass support vector machines for diagnosis of erythemato-squamous diseases. Expert Systems with Applications 35, 1733–1740 (2008)
9. Polat, K., Güneş, S.: A novel hybrid intelligent method based on C4.5 decision tree classifier and one-against-all approach for multi-class classification problems. Expert Systems with Applications 36, 1587–1592 (2009)

10. Übeyli, E.D.: Combined neural networks for diagnosis of erythemato-squamous diseases. Expert Systems with Applications 36, 5107–5112 (2009)
11. Übeyli, E.D., Doğdu, E.: Automatic detection of erythemato-squamous diseases using k-Means clustering. Journal of Medical System 34, 179–184 (2010)
12. Liu, H.W., Sun, J.G., et al.: Feature selection with dynamic mutual information. Pattern Recognition 42, 1330–1339 (2009)
13. Karabatak, M., Ince, M.C.: A new feature selection method based on association rules for diagnosis of erythemato-squamous diseases. Expert Systems with Applications 36, 12500–12505 (2009)
14. Xie, J.Y., Xie, W.X., Wang, C.X., et al.: A novel hybrid feature selection method based on IFSFFS and SVM for the diagnosis of erythemato-squamous diseases. In: JMLR Workshop and Conference Proceedings. Workshop on Applications of Pattern Analysis, vol. 11, pp. 142–151. MIT Press, Windsor (2010)
15. Xie, J.Y., Wang, C.X.: Using support vector machines with a novel hybrid feature selection method for diagnosis of erythemato-squamous diseases. Expert Systems With Applications 38, 5809–5815 (2011)
16. Guyon, I., Elisseeff, A.: An introduction to variable and feature selection. Journal of Machine Learning Research 3, 1157–1182 (2003)
17. Fu, K.S., Min, P.J., Li, T.J.: Feature selection in pattern recognition. IEEE Transactions on Systems Science and Cybernetics SSC 6, 33–39 (1970)
18. Chen, Y.W., Lin, C.J.: Combining SVMs with various feature selection strategies (2005), http://www.csie.ntu.edu.tw/~cjlin/papers/features.pdf
19. Kohavi, R., John, G.: Wrappers for feature selection. Artificial Intelligence 1(2), 273–324 (1997)
20. Blum, A., Langley, P.: Selection of relevant features and examples in machine learning. Artificial Intelligence 1(2), 245–271 (1997)
21. Whitney, A.W.: A direct method of nonparametric measurement selection. IEEE Transactions on Computers 20, 1100–1103 (1971)
22. Marill, T., Green, D.M.: On the effectiveness of receptors in recognition systems. IEEE Transactions on Information Theory IT 9, 11–17 (1963)
23. Pudil, P., Novovicova, J., Kittler, J.: Floating search method in feature selection. Pattern Recognition Letters 15, 119–1254 (1994)

Author Index

Antunes, Cláudia   36

Bruder, Ilvio   13

Chen, Guiqiang   63
Chiang, Stanley   61, 131
Chun, Soon Ae   152
Crull, Katja   25

Di, Z.   76
Du, Min   110

Gao, Xinbo   173
Geller, James   152
Goldschmidt, Leonard   1
Groffen, F.   76

Hansen, David   60
Hao, Dong-mei   100
He, Jing   131
Henriques, Rui   36
Heuer, Andreas   13
Huang, Guangyan   131

Ji, Xiang   152
Jiang, Qingshan   121
Jiang, Weitao   49

Kaba, Djibril   88
Kato, Jien   143
Khazanchi, Deepak   4
Klawonn, Frank   25
Klettke, Meike   13
Kukita, Akiko   25

Larios, E.   76
LeDévédec, S.   76
Lei, Jinhu   173
Li, Yongmin   88
Li, Yurong   110
Liu, Jianjun   63
Liu, Xiaohui   131, 173
Löper, Dortje   13

Okumura, Takashi   164
Owens, Dawn   4

Pessler, Frank   25

Salazar-Gonzalez, Ana   88
Shi, Yong   173
Shu, Libing   49
Steyn, Michael   3

Tateisi, Yuka   164
Tian, Hua   100

Verbeek, F.J.   76

Wang, Liqin   63
Wang, Yu   143
Wang, Zidong   110
Wei, Dan   121
Wei, Yanjie   121
Wu, Huiqin   49
Wu, Song-hong   100

Xie, Juanying   173
Xie, Weixin   173
Xin, Yefei   131

Yan, K.   76
Young, Terry   62
Yu, Xiaodan   4

Zeng, Nianyin   110
Zhang, Hailun   131
Zhang, Hao Lan   49, 131
Zhang, Li   100
Zhang, Yanchun   131
Zhang, Y.   76
Zhao, Jie   100
Zheng, Wei   100
Zhuang, Weiwei   121